I know
what to feed my baby

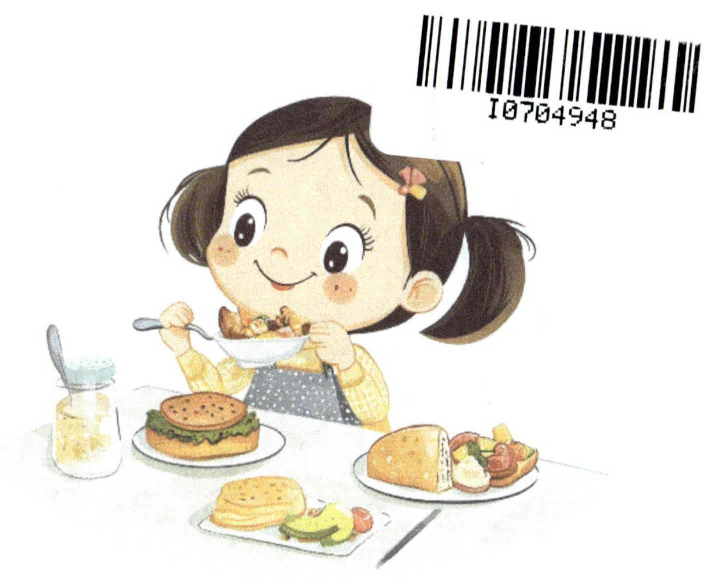

200 healthy and balanced recipes for children

from 1 to 6 years old

VITA KOSTIUK

ISBN: 9798340619105

CONTENTS

ACKNOWLEDGMENTS

This is not a book about healthy eating, and I'm not here to push any feeding plan or lecture you on the benefits or harms of anything! There's already an overload of that information out there! I'm just a mom, and I know that sometimes moms feel tired or scattered and can't think of what to make for breakfast! This is simply a book filled with recipes for feeding your child! Simple and balanced! Just keep it in your kitchen and let it make your life easier!

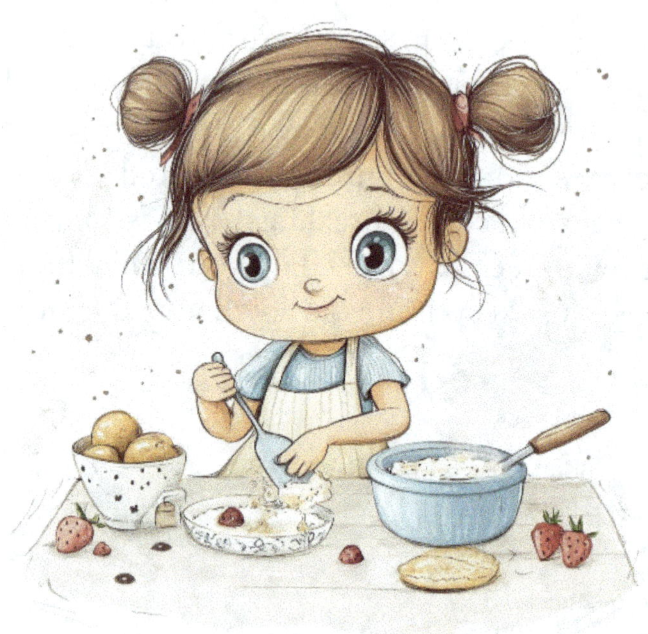

1. Oatmeal with Berries

- **Ingredients:** ½ cup rolled oats, 1 cup milk or water, ¼ cup mixed berries, 1 tsp honey (optional)
- **Preparation:** Cook oats in milk or water until soft. Top with berries and drizzle with honey if desired.

2. Banana Pancakes

- **Ingredients:** 1 ripe banana, 1 egg, ¼ cup flour, 1 tbsp milk
- **Preparation:** Mash the banana and mix with egg, flour, and milk. Cook small pancakes in a non-stick pan until golden.

3. Avocado Toast

- **Ingredients:** ½ avocado, 1 slice whole-grain bread, pinch of salt, cherry tomatoes (optional)
- **Preparation:** Mash avocado with a pinch of salt and spread on toasted bread. Add sliced cherry tomatoes on top.

4. Fruit and Yogurt Parfait

- **Ingredients:** ½ cup plain yogurt, ¼ cup granola, ¼ cup mixed fruits (strawberries, blueberries, etc.)
- **Preparation:** Layer yogurt, granola, and fruits in a glass or bowl.

5. Egg Muffins

- **Ingredients:** 2 eggs, ¼ cup chopped spinach, ¼ cup grated cheese, salt and pepper to taste
- **Preparation:** Whisk eggs with spinach and cheese. Pour into a greased muffin tin and bake at 350°F (175°C) for 15 minutes.

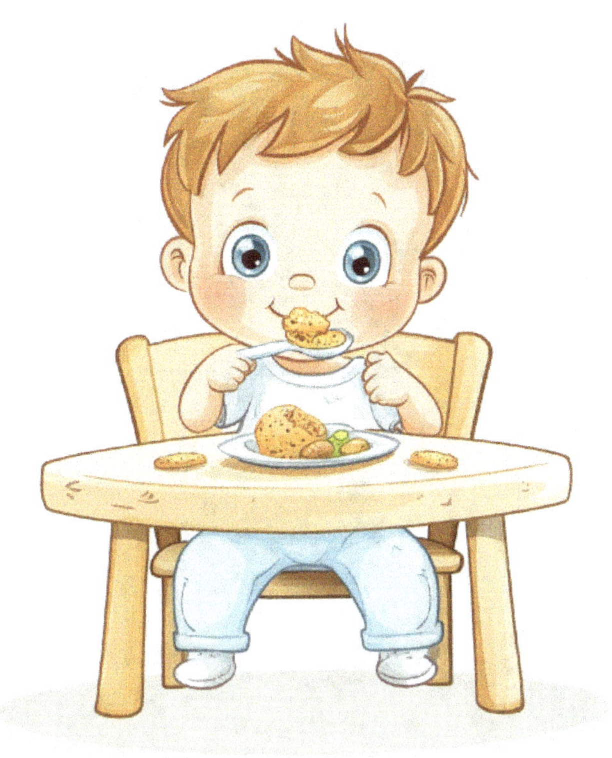

6. Apple Cinnamon Oatmeal

- **Ingredients:** ½ cup rolled oats, 1 apple (diced), 1 tsp cinnamon, 1 cup milk
- **Preparation:** Cook oats and apple in milk. Stir in cinnamon and serve warm.

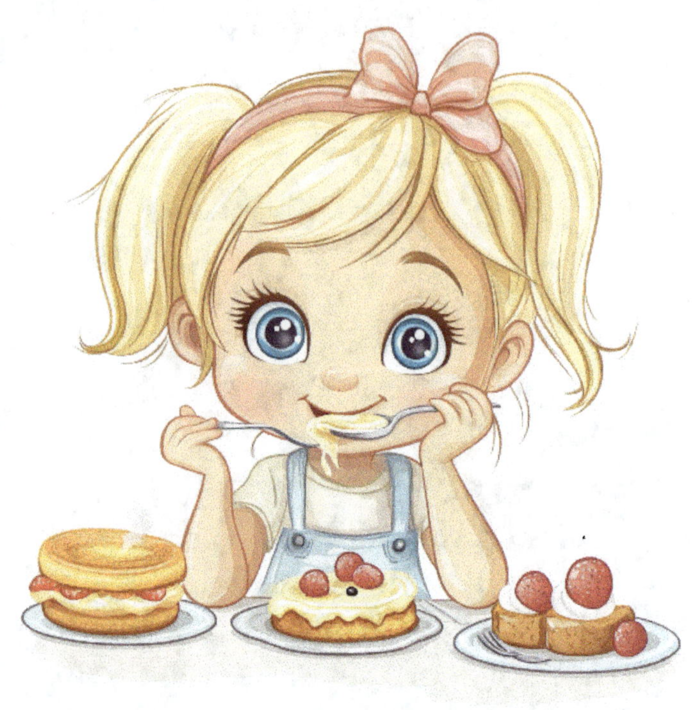

7. Smoothie Bowl

- **Ingredients:** 1 banana, ½ cup frozen berries, ¼ cup yogurt, ¼ cup granola
- **Preparation:** Blend banana, berries, and yogurt until smooth. Pour into a bowl and top with granola.

8. Cheese and Veggie Omelette

- **Ingredients:** 2 eggs, ¼ cup grated cheese, ¼ cup chopped bell peppers, salt and pepper to taste
- **Preparation:** Whisk eggs and pour into a pan. Add cheese and peppers, cook until eggs are set.

9. Whole-Grain Cereal with Milk

- **Ingredients:** 1 cup whole-grain cereal, ½ cup milk, 1 banana (sliced)
- **Preparation:** Serve cereal in a bowl with milk and sliced banana on top.

10. Peanut Butter and Banana Sandwich

- **Ingredients:** 1 slice whole-grain bread, 1 tbsp peanut butter, ½ banana (sliced)
- **Preparation:** Spread peanut butter on bread and top with banana slices.

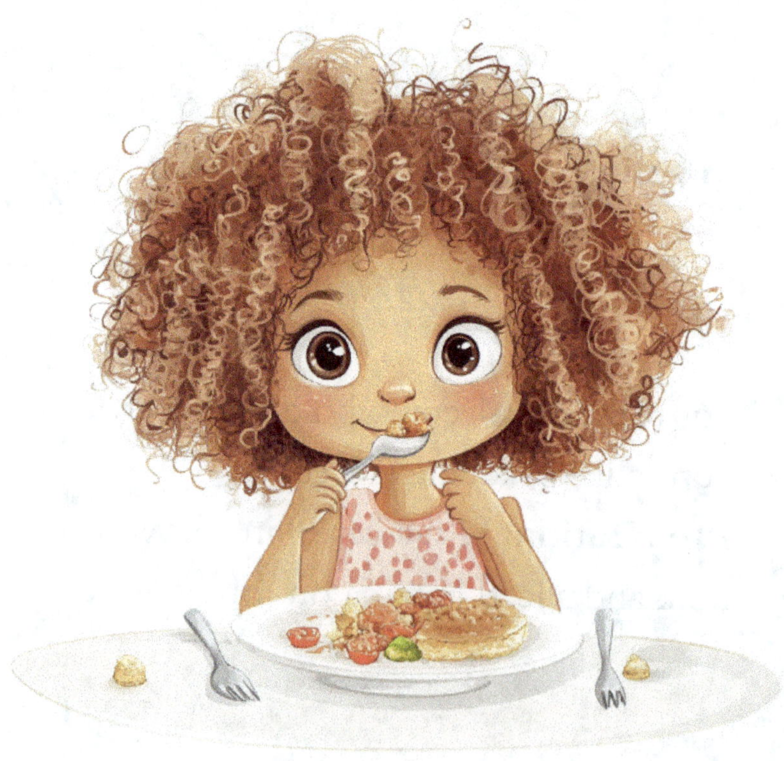

11. Blueberry Muffins

- **Ingredients:** 1 cup flour, ½ cup blueberries, ¼ cup sugar, 1 egg, ¼ cup milk, 1 tsp baking powder
- **Preparation:** Mix ingredients and pour into muffin tin. Bake at 350°F (175°C) for 20 minutes.

12. Greek Yogurt with Honey and Nuts

- **Ingredients:** ½ cup Greek yogurt, 1 tsp honey, 1 tbsp chopped nuts (walnuts, almonds)
- **Preparation:** Mix yogurt with honey and sprinkle nuts on top.

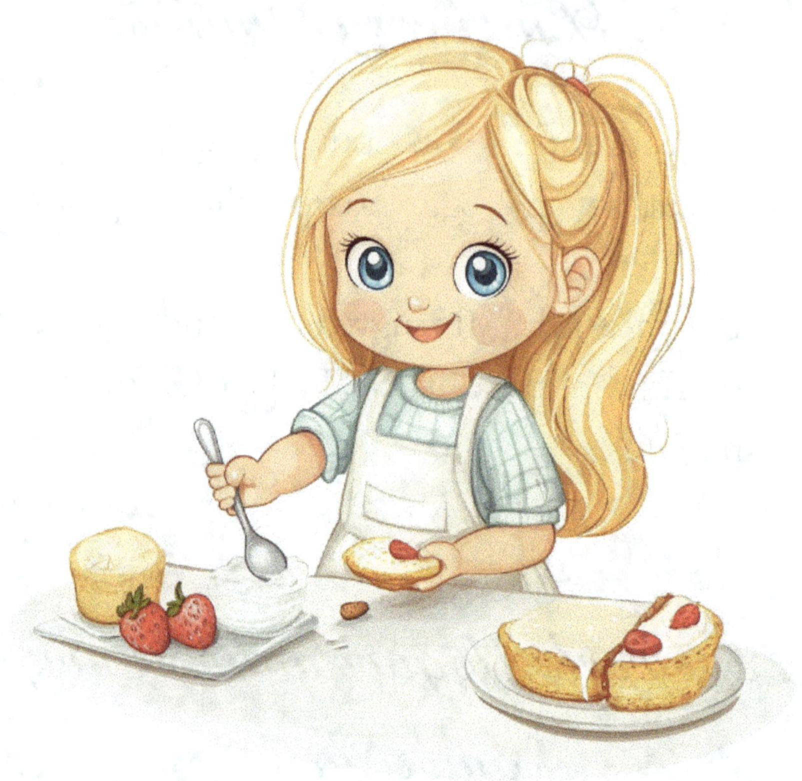

13. Pumpkin Pancakes

- **Ingredients:** ½ cup pumpkin puree, 1 egg, ¼ cup flour, 1 tsp cinnamon
- **Preparation:** Mix all ingredients and cook small pancakes on a non-stick pan.

14. Veggie and Cheese Quesadilla

- **Ingredients:** 1 small whole-grain tortilla, ¼ cup grated cheese, ¼ cup chopped veggies (bell peppers, zucchini)
- **Preparation:** Place cheese and veggies on half of the tortilla, fold, and cook in a pan until cheese melts.

15. Chia Pudding

- **Ingredients:** 2 tbsp chia seeds, ½ cup milk, 1 tsp honey, ¼ cup diced fruit (mango, berries)
- **Preparation:** Mix chia seeds with milk and honey. Let sit overnight and top with fruit in the morning.

16. Scrambled Eggs with Spinach

- **Ingredients:** 2 eggs, ¼ cup chopped spinach, salt and pepper to taste
- **Preparation:** Whisk eggs and cook with spinach until eggs are set.

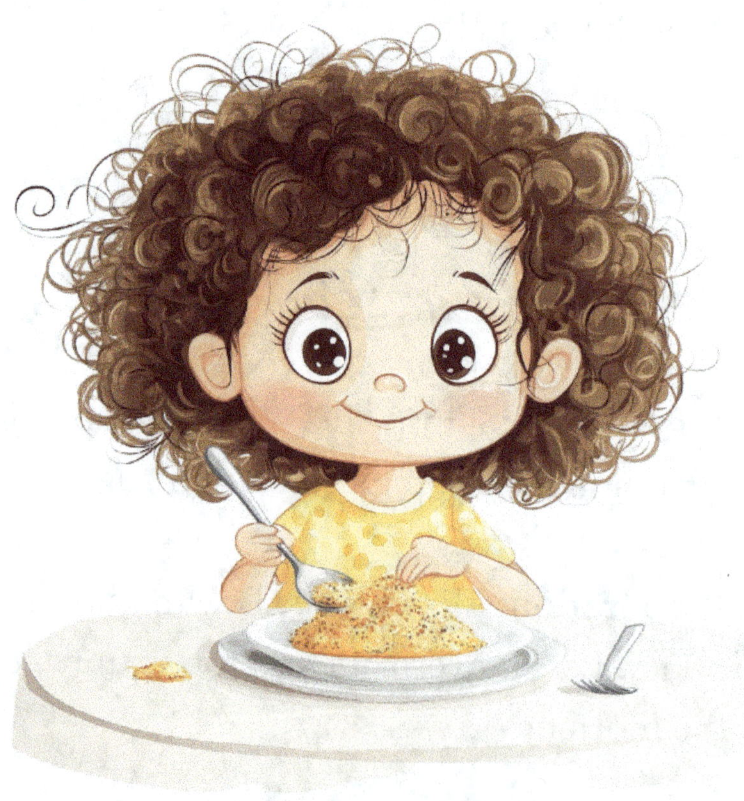

17. Mini Bagels with Cream Cheese and Cucumber

- **Ingredients:** 1 mini whole-grain bagel, 1 tbsp cream cheese, 4 slices cucumber
- **Preparation:** Spread cream cheese on bagel and top with cucumber slices.

18. Carrot and Apple Muffins

- **Ingredients:** 1 cup flour, 1 carrot (grated), 1 apple (grated), ¼ cup sugar, 1 egg, ¼ cup milk, 1 tsp baking powder
- **Preparation:** Mix all ingredients and pour into muffin tin. Bake at 350°F (175°C) for 20 minutes.

19. Fruit Smoothie

- **Ingredients:** 1 banana, ½ cup frozen berries, ¼ cup yogurt, ½ cup milk
- **Preparation:** Blend all ingredients until smooth.

20. Egg-in-a-Hole

- **Ingredients:** 1 slice whole-grain bread, 1 egg, 1 tsp butter
- **Preparation:** Cut a hole in the center of the bread. Cook in a pan with butter, crack egg into the hole, and cook until egg is set.

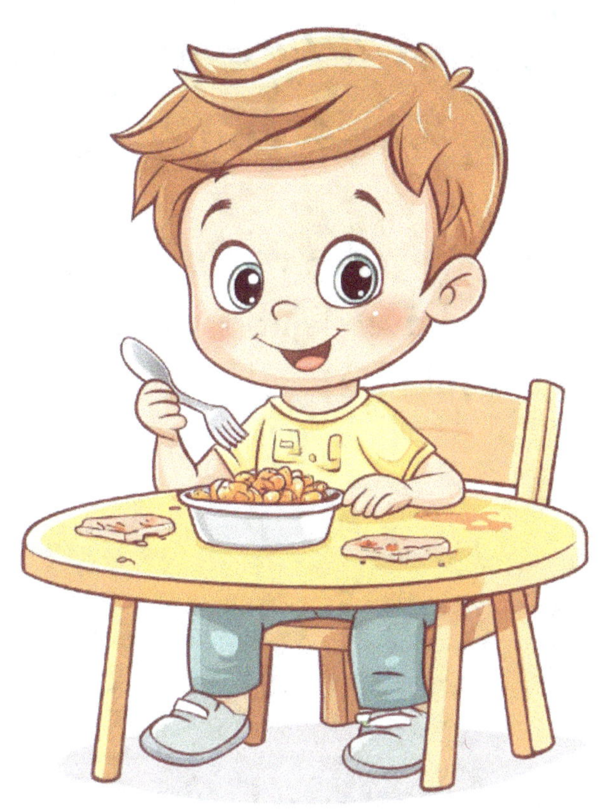

21. Zucchini Fritters

- **Ingredients:** 1 small zucchini (grated), 1 egg, ¼ cup flour, salt and pepper to taste
- **Preparation:** Mix ingredients and cook small fritters in a non-stick pan until golden.

22. Yogurt with Granola and Fresh Fruit

- **Ingredients:** ½ cup yogurt, ¼ cup granola, ¼ cup diced fresh fruit (kiwi, apple)
- **Preparation:** Layer yogurt, granola, and fruit in a bowl.

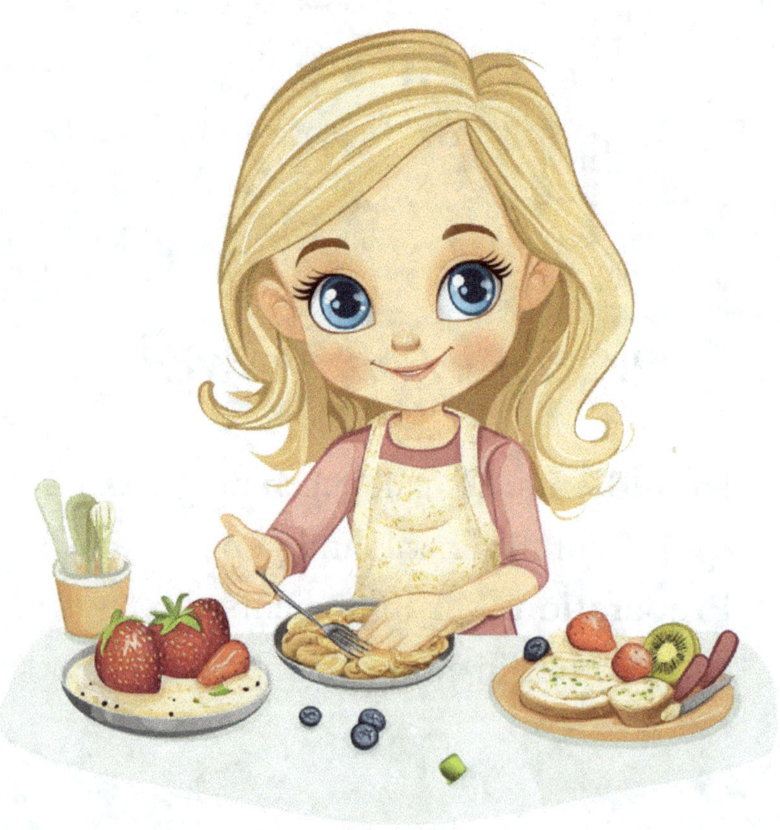

23. Cottage Cheese with Peaches

- **Ingredients:** ½ cup cottage cheese, ½ cup diced peaches
- **Preparation:** Mix cottage cheese with peaches and serve.

24. Spinach and Cheese Toast

- **Ingredients:** 1 slice whole-grain bread, ¼ cup chopped spinach, ¼ cup grated cheese
- **Preparation:** Top bread with spinach and cheese, then toast until cheese melts.

25. Banana Oat Cookies

- **Ingredients:** 1 ripe banana, ½ cup oats, 1 tbsp honey (optional)
- **Preparation:** Mash banana and mix with oats. Form small cookies and bake at 350°F (175°C) for 15 minutes.

26. Pear and Cinnamon Porridge

- **Ingredients:** ½ cup rolled oats, 1 pear (diced), 1 tsp cinnamon, 1 cup milk
- **Preparation:** Cook oats and pear in milk. Stir in cinnamon and serve warm.

27. Sweet Potato and Apple Hash

- **Ingredients:** 1 small sweet potato (diced), 1 apple (diced), 1 tbsp butter
- **Preparation:** Cook sweet potato and apple in butter until soft.

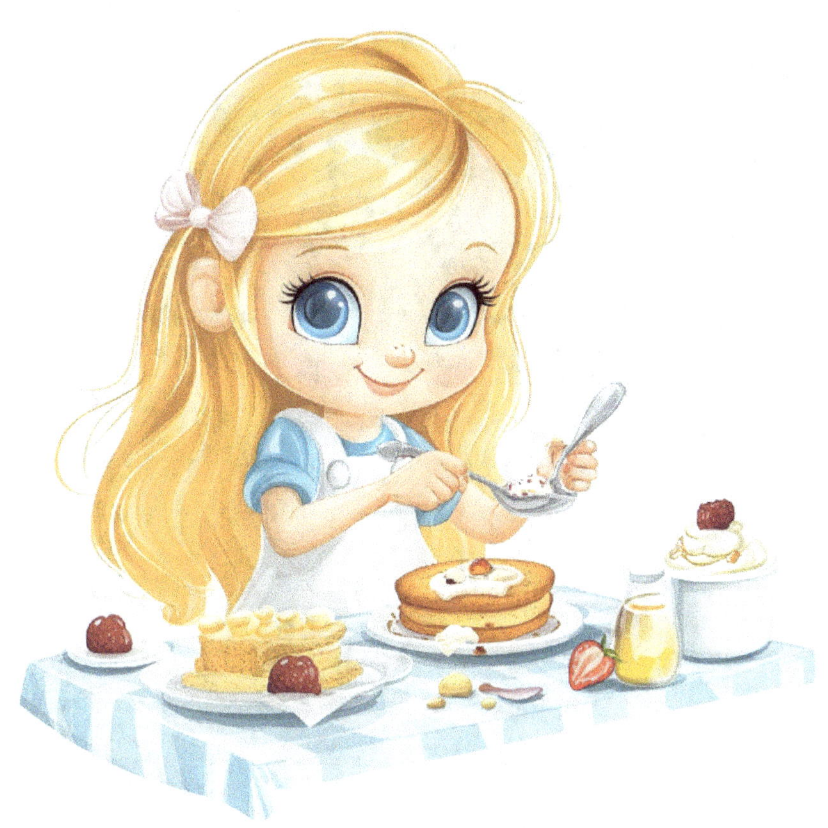

28. Cucumber and Cream Cheese Sandwich

- **Ingredients:** 1 slice whole-grain bread, 1 tbsp cream cheese, 4 slices cucumber
- **Preparation:** Spread cream cheese on bread and top with cucumber slices.

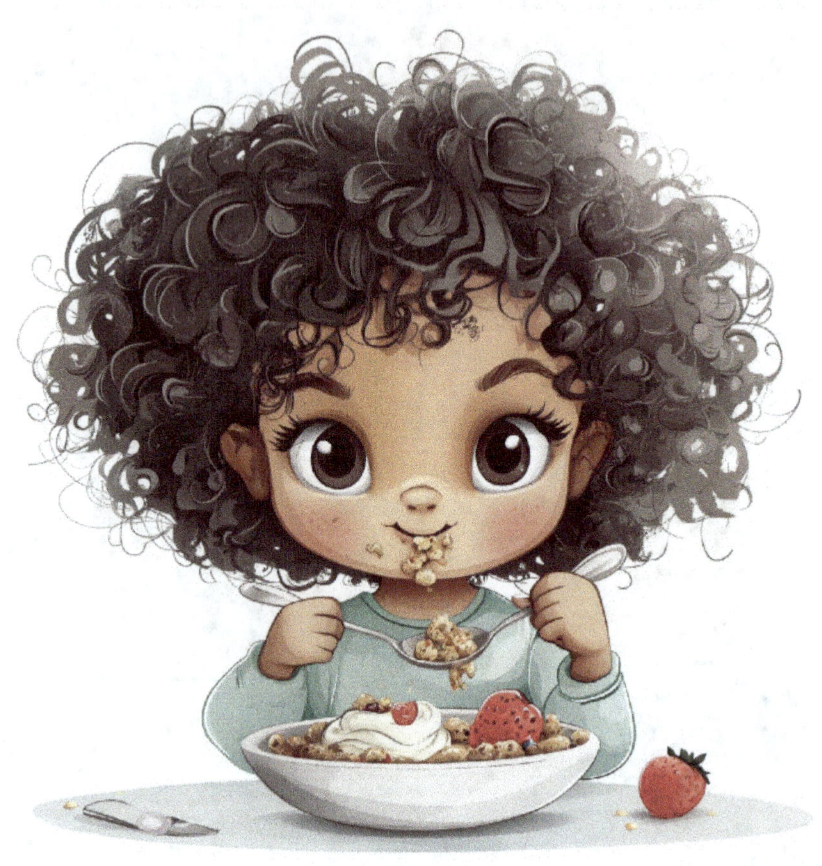

29. Egg and Cheese Breakfast Burrito

- **Ingredients:** 1 small whole-grain tortilla, 1 egg, ¼ cup grated cheese
- **Preparation:** Scramble egg and place in tortilla with cheese. Roll up and cook in a pan until cheese melts.

30. Pumpkin Oatmeal

- **Ingredients:** ½ cup rolled oats, ¼ cup pumpkin puree, 1 tsp cinnamon, 1 cup milk
- **Preparation:** Cook oats in milk, stir in pumpkin and cinnamon.

31. Berry and Yogurt Popsicles

- **Ingredients:** 1 cup yogurt, ½ cup mixed berries, 1 tsp honey (optional)
- **Preparation:** Blend yogurt and berries. Pour into popsicle molds and freeze.

32. French Toast Sticks

- **Ingredients:** 1 slice whole-grain bread, 1 egg, ¼ cup milk, 1 tsp cinnamon
- **Preparation:** Cut bread into sticks. Dip in egg and milk mixture, sprinkle with cinnamon, and cook in a pan until golden.

33. Vegetable Pancakes

- **Ingredients:** 1 small carrot (grated), 1 small zucchini (grated), 1 egg, ¼ cup flour
- **Preparation:** Mix ingredients and cook small pancakes in a non-stick pan until golden.

34. Banana and Almond Butter Wrap

- **Ingredients:** 1 small whole-grain tortilla, 1 tbsp almond butter, ½ banana (sliced)
- **Preparation:** Spread almond butter on tortilla and top with banana slices. Roll up and serve.

35. Cinnamon Apple Slices

- **Ingredients:** 1 apple (sliced), 1 tsp cinnamon
- **Preparation:** Sprinkle apple slices with cinnamon and serve.

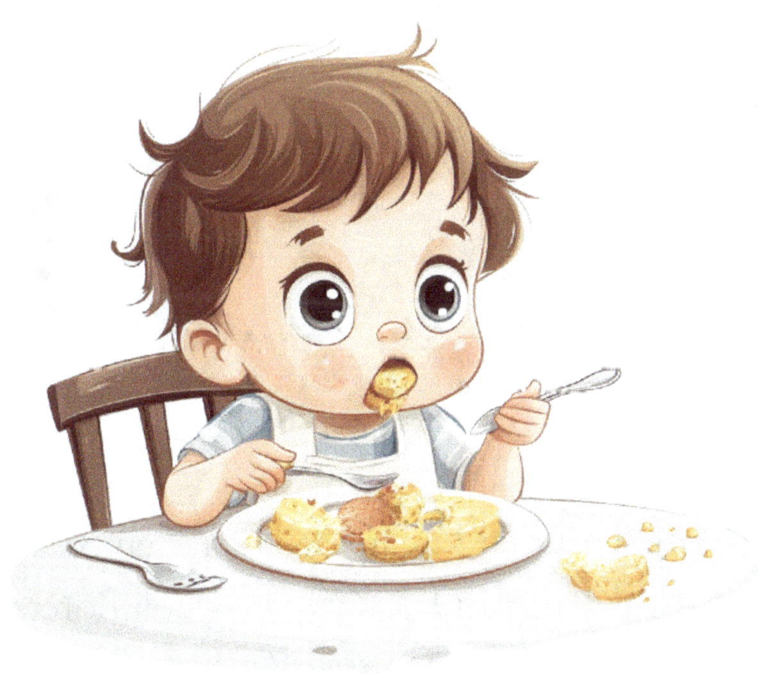

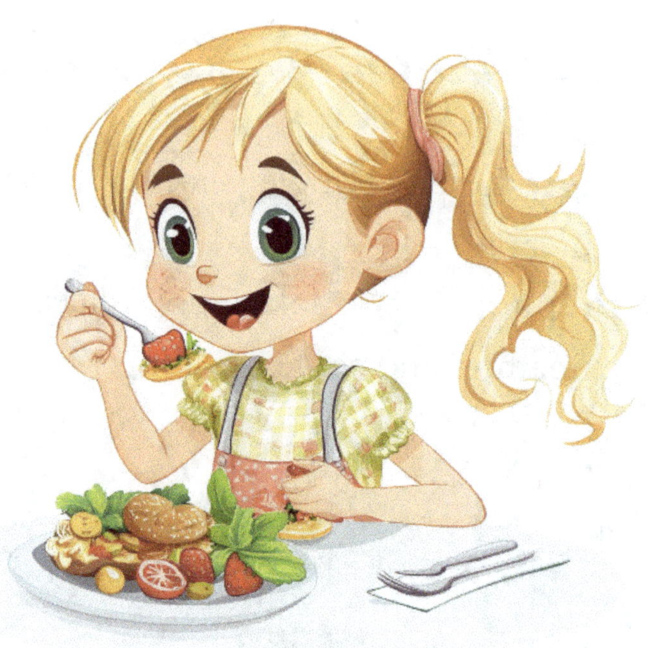

1. Chicken and Vegetable Stir-Fry

- **Ingredients:** ½ cup diced chicken breast, ¼ cup diced carrots, ¼ cup broccoli florets, 1 tbsp olive oil, 1 tsp soy sauce

- **Preparation:** Cook chicken in olive oil until browned. Add vegetables and soy sauce, sauté until tender.

2. *Macaroni and Cheese with Peas*

- **Ingredients:** ½ cup whole-grain macaroni, ¼ cup shredded cheese, ¼ cup frozen peas, 1 tbsp butter
- **Preparation:** Cook macaroni and peas together. Drain and stir in butter and cheese until melted.
-

3. *Turkey and Avocado Wrap*

- **Ingredients:** 1 small whole-grain tortilla, 2 slices turkey breast, ¼ avocado (sliced), 1 tbsp cream cheese
- **Preparation:** Spread cream cheese on tortilla, add turkey and avocado slices, and roll up.

4. Vegetable Soup

- **Ingredients:** ½ cup diced carrots, ½ cup diced potatoes, ¼ cup green beans, 2 cups vegetable broth
- **Preparation:** Boil vegetables in broth until tender. Puree for younger children or serve as is.

5. Mini Meatballs with Spaghetti

- **Ingredients:** ¼ lb ground beef or turkey, ¼ cup breadcrumbs, 1 egg, ½ cup whole-grain spaghetti, ¼ cup marinara sauce
- **Preparation:** Mix meat with breadcrumbs and egg, form small meatballs, and bake at 350°F (175°C) for 15 minutes. Serve over spaghetti with marinara sauce.

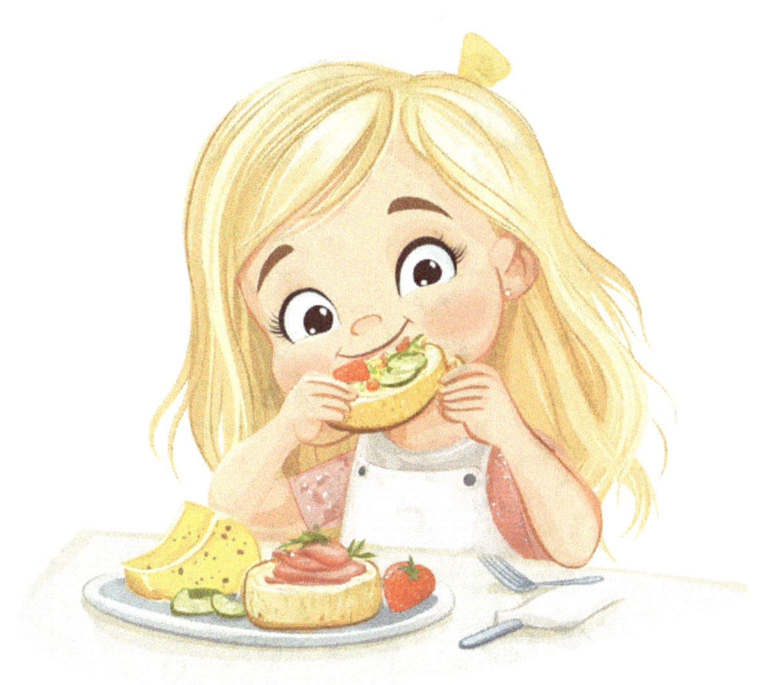

6. Baked Sweet Potato with Broccoli

- **Ingredients:** 1 small sweet potato, ¼ cup steamed broccoli, 1 tbsp butter
- **Preparation:** Bake sweet potato at 375°F (190°C) for 45 minutes. Split open and top with broccoli and butter.

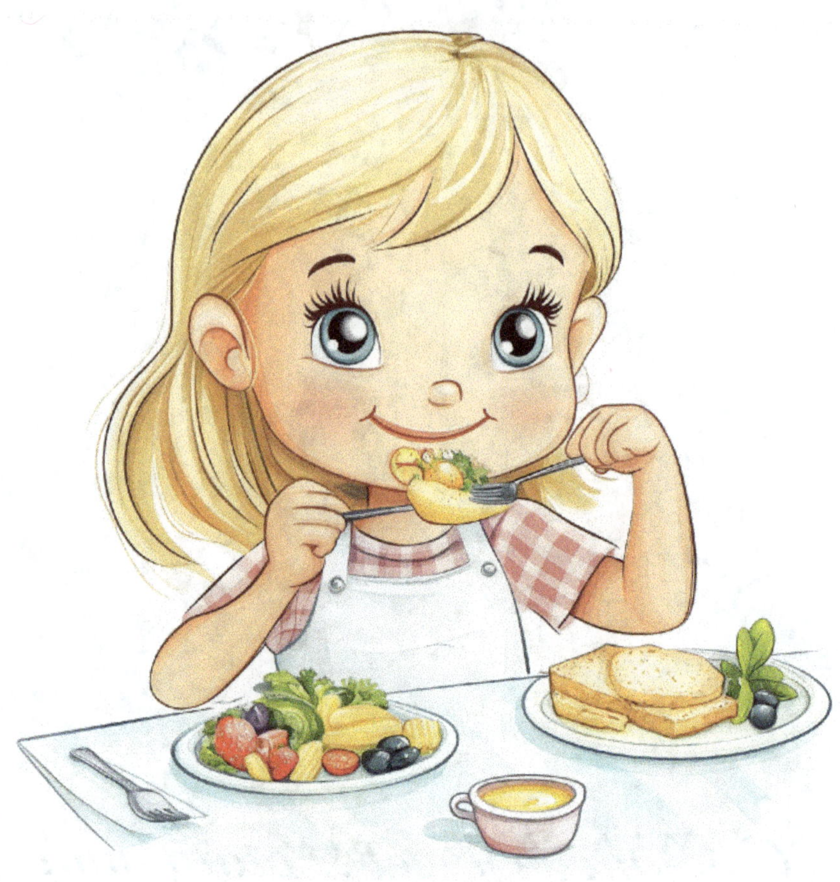

7. Grilled Cheese and Tomato Sandwich

- **Ingredients:** 2 slices whole-grain bread, 1 slice cheese, 2 slices tomato, 1 tbsp butter
- **Preparation:** Assemble sandwich with cheese and tomato. Cook in a pan with butter until golden brown.

8. Chicken and Rice Casserole

- **Ingredients:** ½ cup cooked rice, ¼ cup diced chicken, ¼ cup mixed vegetables, 1 tbsp cream of chicken soup
- **Preparation:** Mix ingredients and bake at 350°F (175°C) for 20 minutes.

9. Lentil Stew

- **Ingredients:** ½ cup lentils, ¼ cup diced carrots, ¼ cup diced potatoes, 2 cups vegetable broth
- **Preparation:** Simmer lentils and vegetables in broth until soft. Puree for younger children if needed.

10. Egg Salad Sandwich

- **Ingredients:** 1 boiled egg, 1 tbsp mayonnaise, 1 slice whole-grain bread, 1 lettuce leaf
- **Preparation:** Mash egg with mayonnaise, spread on bread, and add lettuce.

11. Fish Sticks with Mashed Potatoes

- **Ingredients:** 2-3 fish sticks, 1 small potato, 1 tbsp butter, ¼ cup milk
- **Preparation:** Bake fish sticks according to package instructions. Boil and mash potato with butter and milk.

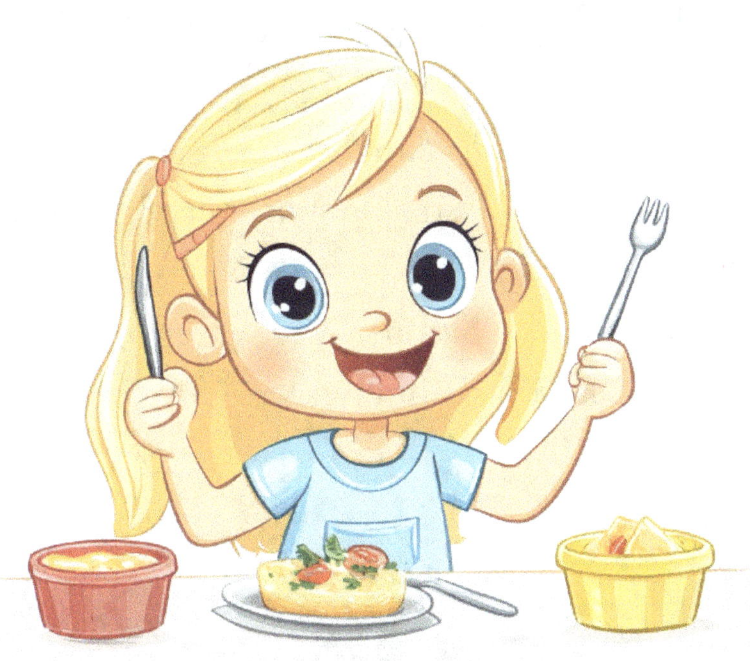

12. Vegetable Quesadilla

- **Ingredients:** 1 small whole-grain tortilla, ¼ cup shredded cheese, ¼ cup diced bell peppers and zucchini
- **Preparation:** Place cheese and vegetables on one half of the tortilla, fold, and cook in a pan until cheese melts.

13. Chicken and Corn Soup

- **Ingredients:** ½ cup diced chicken, ¼ cup corn kernels, 1 small potato (diced), 2 cups chicken broth
- **Preparation:** Simmer chicken, corn, and potato in broth until tender

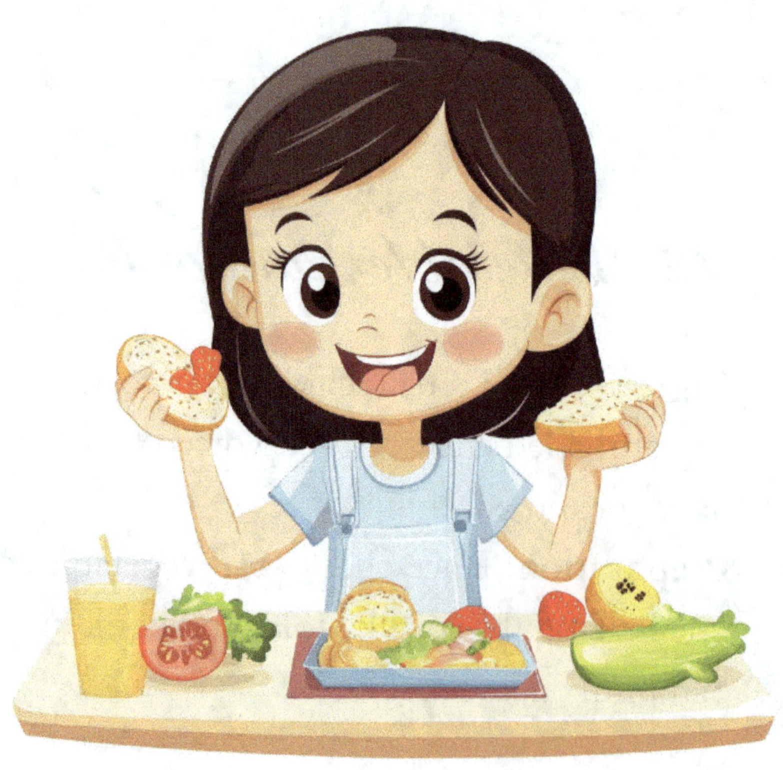

14. Pasta Primavera

- **Ingredients:** ½ cup whole-grain pasta, ¼ cup diced zucchini, ¼ cup cherry tomatoes (halved), 1 tbsp olive oil
- **Preparation:** Cook pasta, sauté vegetables in olive oil, and toss with pasta.

15. Spinach and Cheese Omelette

- **Ingredients:** 2 eggs, ¼ cup chopped spinach, ¼ cup shredded cheese, salt to taste
- **Preparation:** Whisk eggs, pour into a pan, add spinach and cheese, and cook until eggs are set.

16. Beef and Vegetable Skewers

- **Ingredients:** ¼ lb beef (cubed), ¼ cup bell peppers (cubed), ¼ cup zucchini (cubed)
- **Preparation:** Thread beef and vegetables onto skewers and grill until meat is cooked through.

17. Chicken and Apple Salad

- **Ingredients:** ½ cup diced chicken, ½ apple (diced), 1 tbsp yogurt, 1 tsp lemon juice
- **Preparation:** Mix chicken and apple with yogurt and lemon juice.

18. Broccoli and Cheese Baked Potatoes

- **Ingredients:** 1 small potato, ¼ cup steamed broccoli, ¼ cup shredded cheese
- **Preparation:** Bake potato at 375°F (190°C) for 45 minutes. Split open and top with broccoli and cheese.

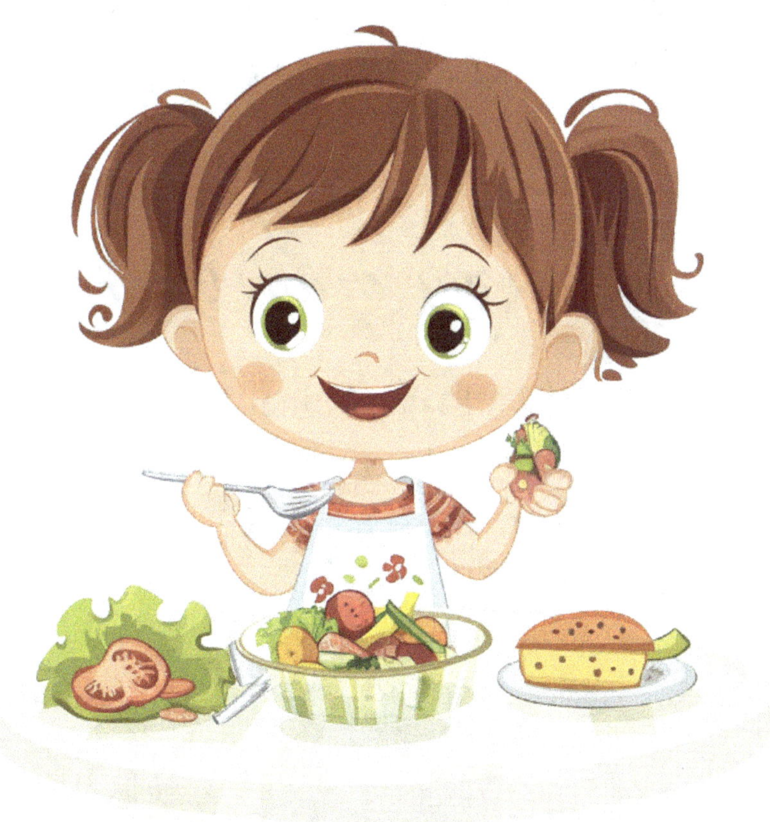

19. Turkey and Veggie Roll-Ups

- **Ingredients:** 2 slices turkey breast, ¼ cup diced vegetables (carrots, cucumbers), 1 tbsp cream cheese
- **Preparation:** Spread cream cheese on turkey slices, add vegetables, and roll up.

20. Vegetarian Chili

- **Ingredients:** ½ cup kidney beans, ¼ cup diced tomatoes, ¼ cup corn, ¼ cup diced bell peppers, 1 tsp chili powder
- **Preparation:** Simmer all ingredients together until flavors blend.

21. Chicken and Cheese Pinwheels

- **Ingredients:** 1 small whole-grain tortilla, 2 slices chicken breast, ¼ cup shredded cheese, 1 tbsp cream cheese
- **Preparation:** Spread cream cheese on tortilla, add chicken and cheese, roll up, and slice into pinwheels.

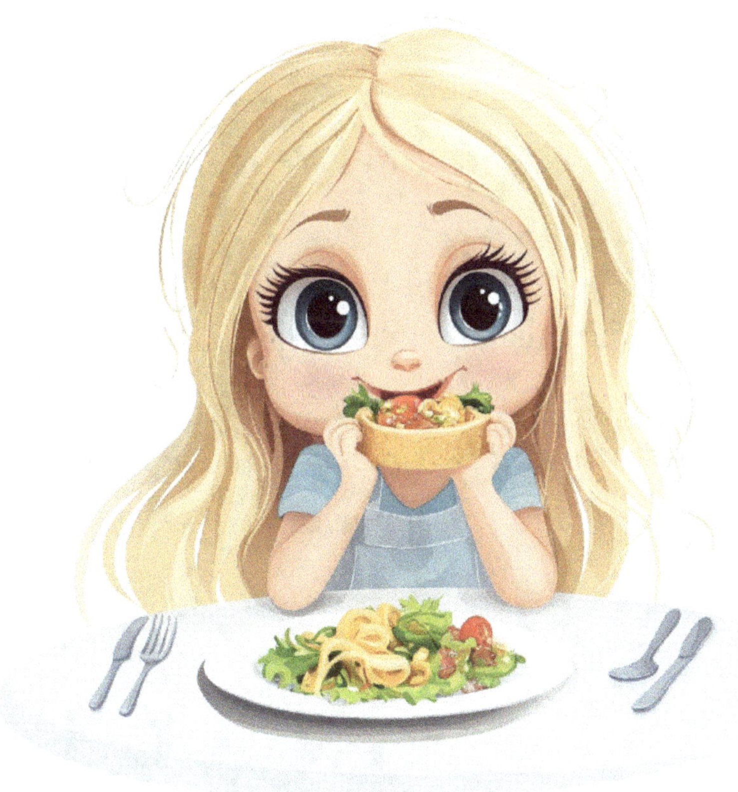

22. *Stuffed Bell Peppers*

- **Ingredients:** 1 small bell pepper, ¼ cup cooked rice, ¼ cup ground turkey or beef, 2 tbsp tomato sauce
- **Preparation:** Mix rice, meat, and tomato sauce. Stuff into bell pepper and bake at 350°F (175°C) for 20 minutes.

23. *Chicken and Avocado Salad*

- **Ingredients:** ½ cup diced chicken, ¼ avocado (sliced), 1 tbsp olive oil, 1 tsp lemon juice
- **Preparation:** Mix chicken and avocado with olive oil and lemon juice.

24. Mini Pizzas

- **Ingredients:** 1 small whole-grain pita, 2 tbsp tomato sauce, ¼ cup shredded cheese, ¼ cup diced vegetables
- **Preparation:** Spread sauce on pita, add cheese and vegetables, and bake at 350°F (175°C) for 10 minutes.

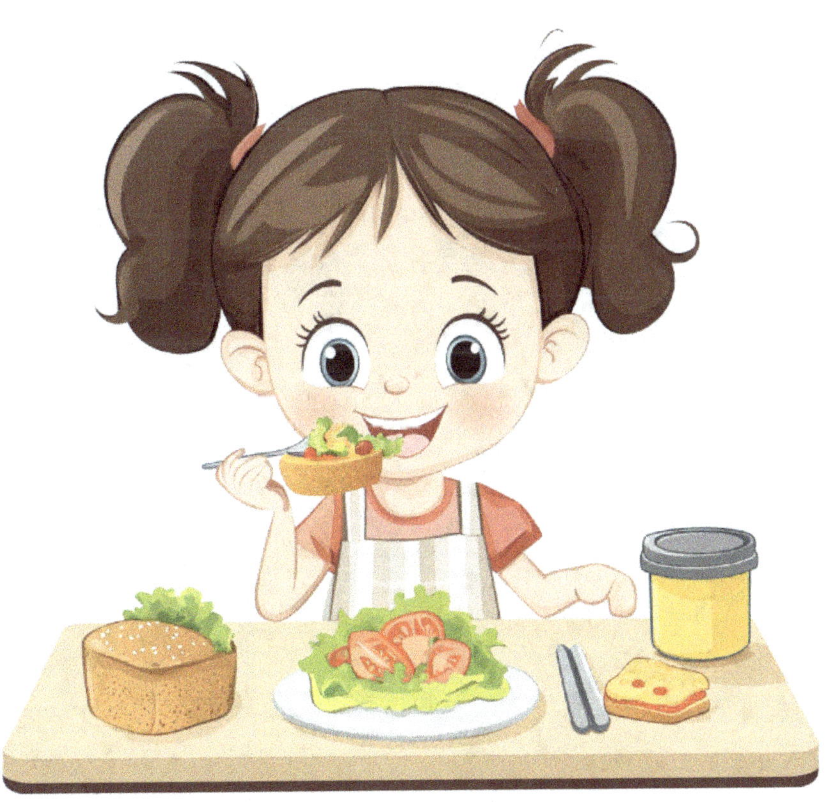

25. Carrot and Lentil Soup

- **Ingredients:** ½ cup red lentils, 2 carrots (sliced), 1 small onion (diced), 2 cups vegetable broth
- **Preparation:** Simmer all ingredients until lentils and carrots are soft. Puree for younger children if needed.

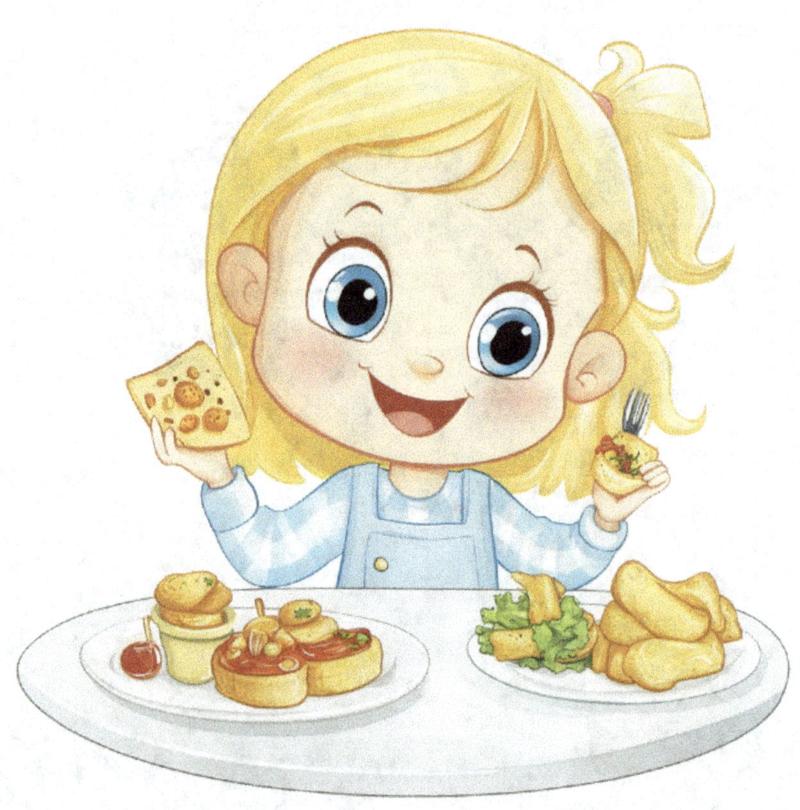

26. Chicken Noodle Soup

- **Ingredients:** ½ cup diced chicken, ¼ cup whole-grain noodles, ¼ cup diced carrots and celery, 2 cups chicken broth
- **Preparation:** Cook chicken, noodles, and vegetables in broth until tender.

27. Rice and Bean Burrito

- **Ingredients:** 1 small whole-grain tortilla, ¼ cup cooked rice, ¼ cup black beans, 2 tbsp shredded cheese
- **Preparation:** Fill tortilla with rice, beans, and cheese, then roll up.

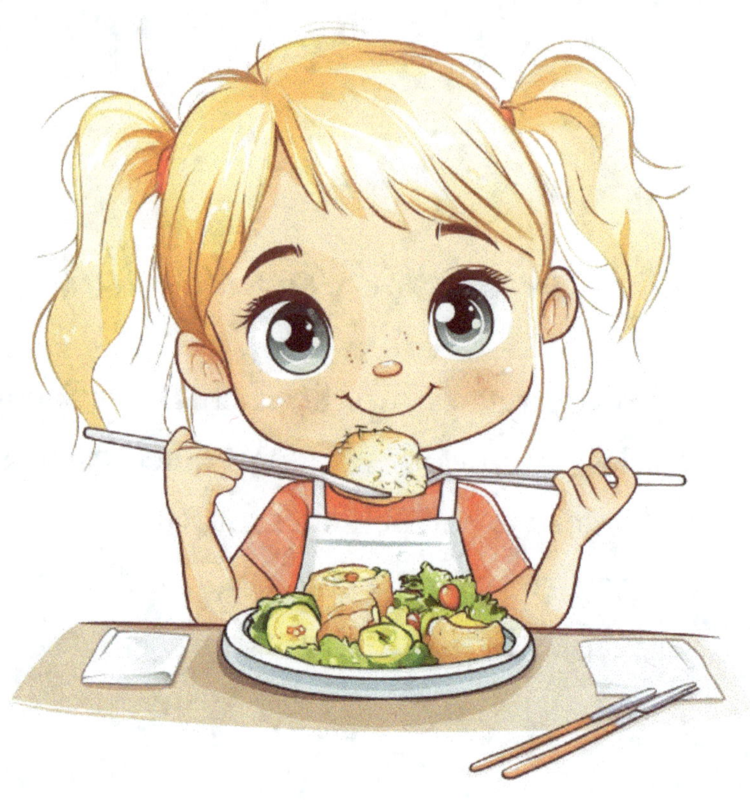

28. Vegetable Risotto

- **Ingredients:** ½ cup Arborio rice, ¼ cup diced zucchini, ¼ cup diced carrots, 2 cups vegetable broth, 1 tbsp butter
- **Preparation:** Cook rice in broth, stirring frequently. Add vegetables halfway through cooking. Stir in butter before serving.

29. Grilled Chicken and Veggie Kabobs

- **Ingredients:** ¼ lb chicken breast (cubed), ¼ cup bell peppers (cubed), ¼ cup zucchini (cubed)
- **Preparation:** Thread chicken and vegetables onto skewers and grill until cooked through.

30. Tomato and Cheese Sandwich

- **Ingredients:** 2 slices whole-grain bread, 1 slice cheese, 2 slices tomato, 1 tbsp hummus
- **Preparation:** Spread hummus on bread, add cheese and tomato, and assemble sandwich.

31. Chicken and Broccoli Pasta

- **Ingredients:** ½ cup whole-grain pasta, ¼ cup diced chicken, ¼ cup steamed broccoli, 1 tbsp olive oil
- **Preparation:** Cook pasta, sauté chicken and broccoli in olive oil, and toss with pasta.

32. Vegetable and Cheese Frittata

- **Ingredients:** 2 eggs, ¼ cup diced vegetables (zucchini, bell peppers), ¼ cup shredded cheese, salt to taste
- **Preparation:** Whisk eggs, add vegetables and cheese, and bake at 350°F (175°C) for 15 minutes.

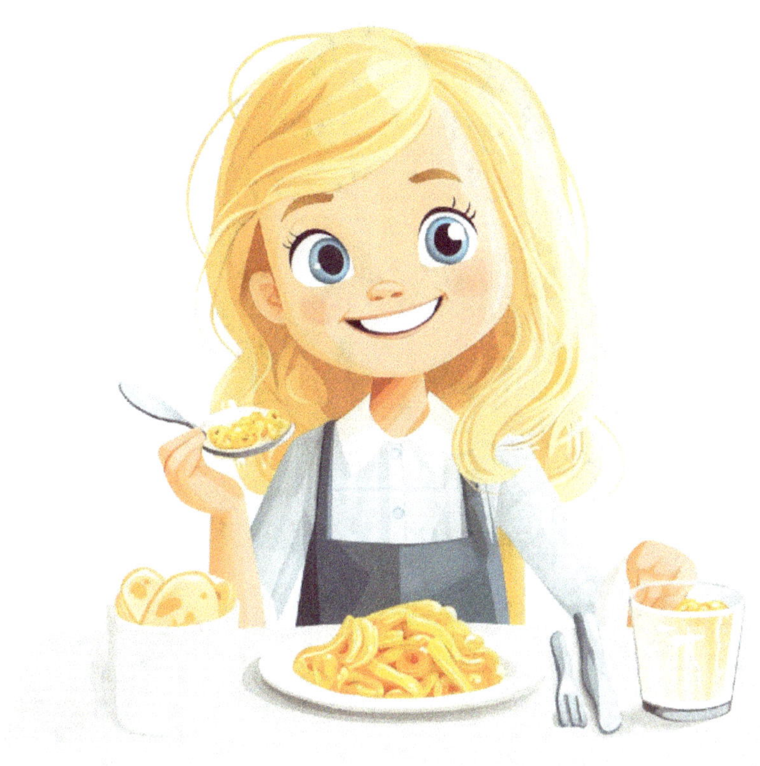

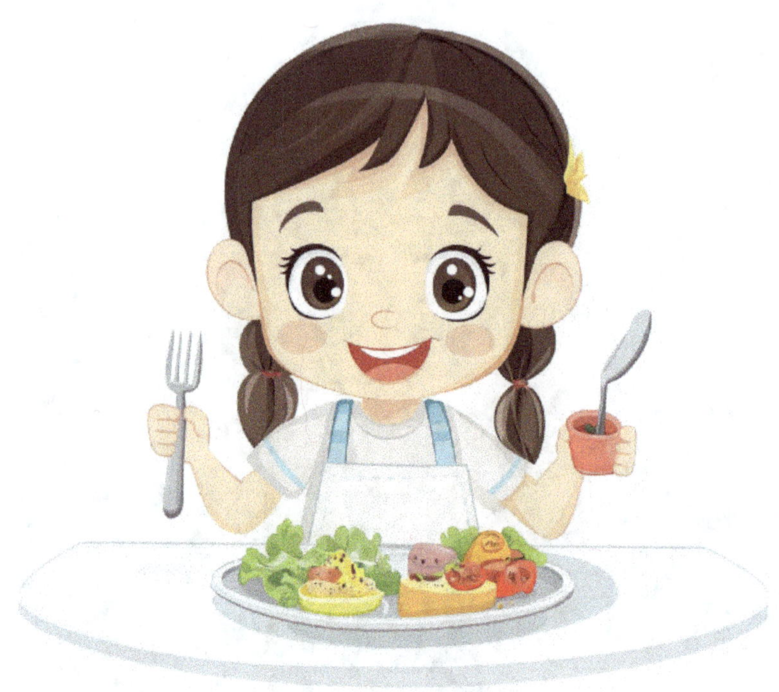

1. Cheese and Veggie Omelette

- **Ingredients:** 2 eggs, ¼ cup chopped spinach, ¼ cup grated cheese, salt to taste
- **Preparation:** Whisk eggs, pour into a pan, add spinach and cheese, and cook until eggs are set.

2. Banana Oat Pancakes

- **Ingredients:** 1 ripe banana, 1 egg, ¼ cup rolled oats, ¼ tsp cinnamon
- **Preparation:** Mash banana, mix with egg, oats, and cinnamon. Cook small pancakes on a non-stick pan until golden.

3. Mini Veggie Frittatas

- **Ingredients:** 2 eggs, ¼ cup diced vegetables (bell peppers, spinach), ¼ cup shredded cheese
- **Preparation:** Mix eggs, veggies, and cheese. Pour into a greased muffin tin and bake at 350°F (175°C) for 15 minutes.

4. Avocado Toast with Boiled Egg

- **Ingredients:** ½ avocado, 1 slice whole-grain bread, 1 boiled egg, pinch of salt
- **Preparation:** Mash avocado and spread on toast. Slice the boiled egg and place on top, sprinkle with salt.

5. Yogurt and Fruit Parfait

- **Ingredients:** ½ cup plain yogurt, ¼ cup granola, ¼ cup mixed berries
- **Preparation:** Layer yogurt, granola, and berries in a bowl or glass.

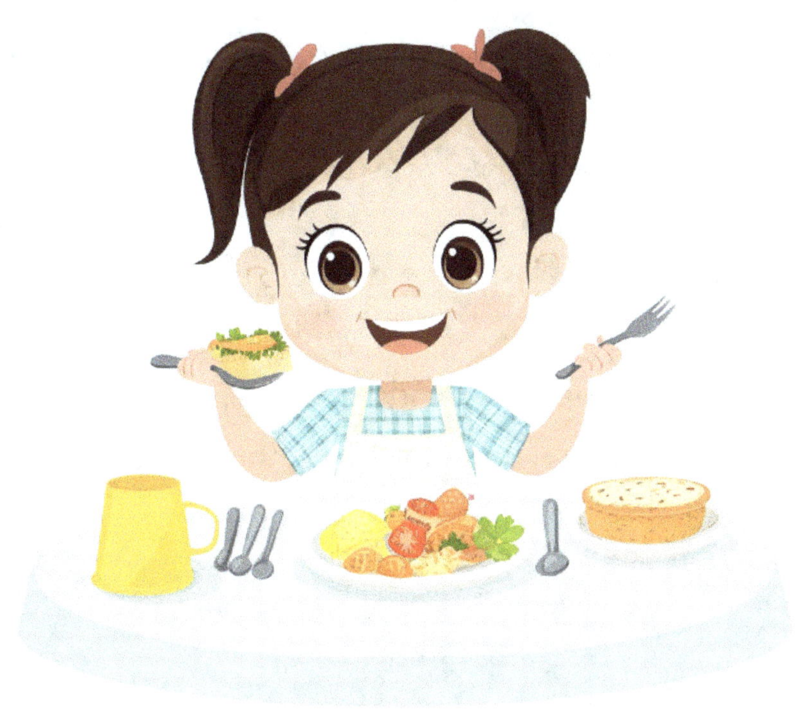

6. Cheese Quesadilla

- **Ingredients:** 1 small whole-grain tortilla, ¼ cup shredded cheese, ¼ cup diced tomatoes
- **Preparation:** Place cheese and tomatoes on one half of the tortilla, fold, and cook in a pan until cheese melts.

7. Banana and Peanut Butter Sandwich

- **Ingredients:** 1 slice whole-grain bread, 1 tbsp peanut butter, ½ banana (sliced)
- **Preparation:** Spread peanut butter on bread, add banana slices, and fold the bread in half.

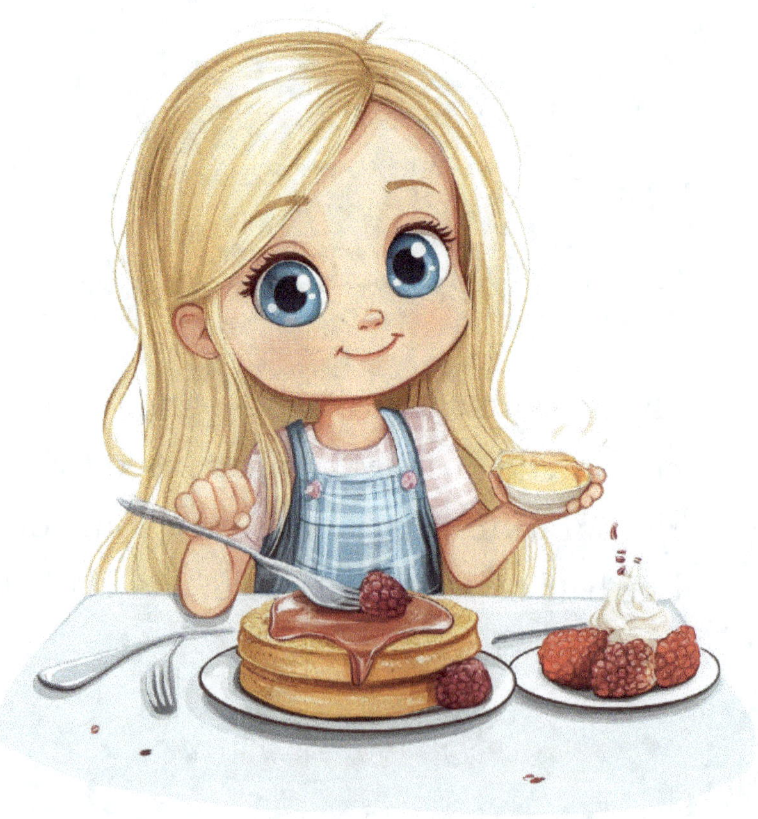

8. Blueberry Muffins

- **Ingredients:** 1 cup whole wheat flour, ½ cup blueberries, ¼ cup sugar, 1 egg, ¼ cup milk, 1 tsp baking powder
- **Preparation:** Mix ingredients and pour into a muffin tin. Bake at 350°F (175°C) for 20 minutes.

9. Apple Cinnamon Oatmeal

- **Ingredients:** ½ cup rolled oats, 1 apple (diced), 1 tsp cinnamon, 1 cup milk or water
- **Preparation:** Cook oats with diced apple in milk or water, stir in cinnamon before serving.

10. Spinach and Cheese Stuffed Mini Bagels

- **Ingredients:** 2 mini whole-grain bagels, ¼ cup chopped spinach, ¼ cup shredded cheese
- **Preparation:** Mix spinach and cheese, then stuff into sliced bagels. Toast until cheese melts.

11. Fruit Smoothie Bowl

- **Ingredients:** 1 banana, ½ cup frozen berries, ¼ cup plain yogurt, ¼ cup granola
- **Preparation:** Blend banana, berries, and yogurt until smooth. Pour into a bowl and top with granola.

12. Egg and Cheese Breakfast Burrito

- **Ingredients:** 1 small whole-grain tortilla, 2 eggs, ¼ cup shredded cheese, 1 tbsp salsa (optional)
- **Preparation:** Scramble eggs, place in tortilla with cheese and salsa, and roll up.

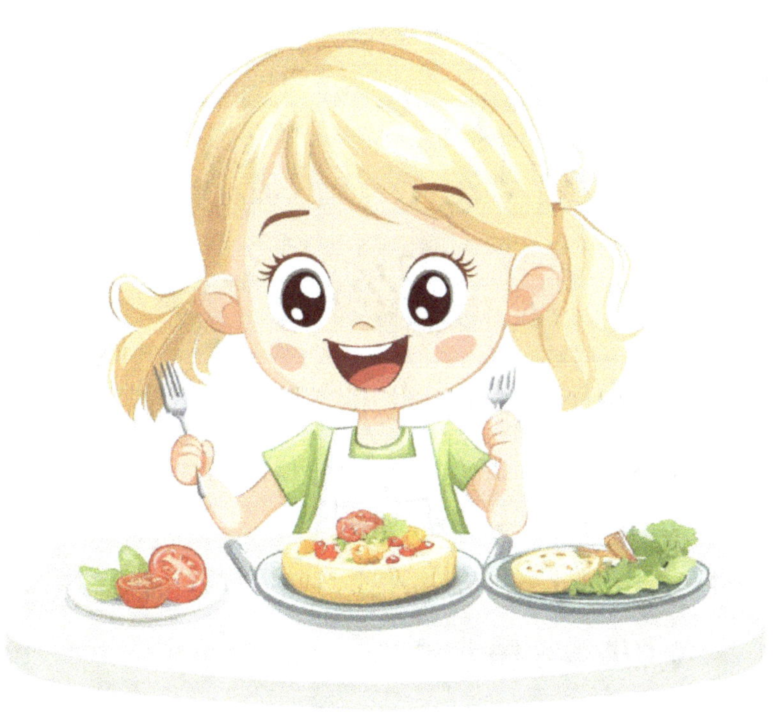

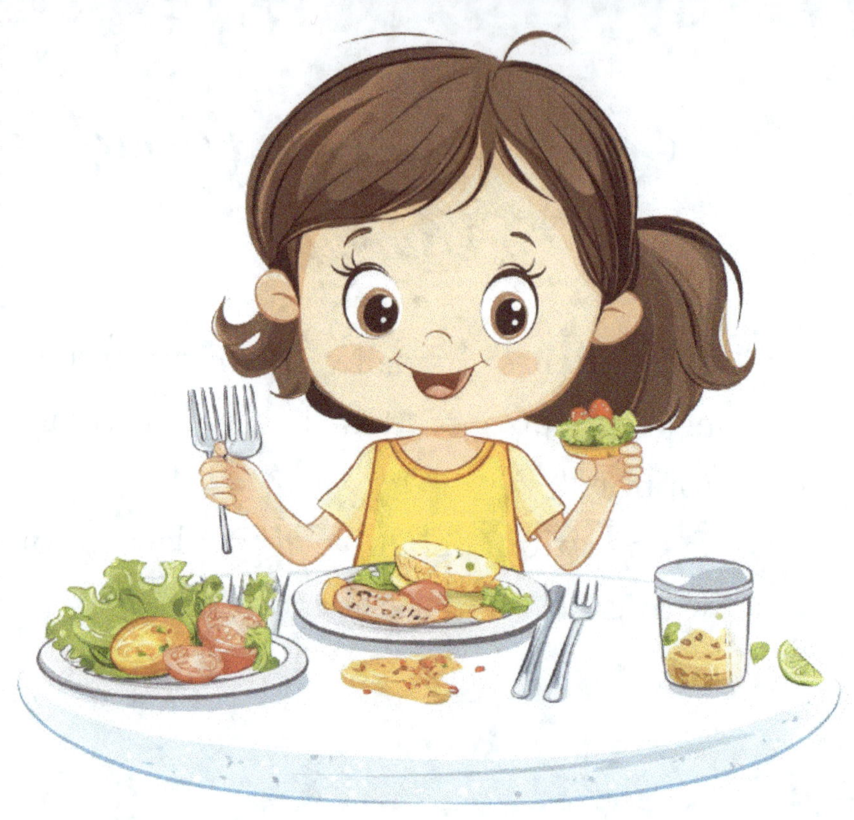

13. Vegetable and Cheese Roll-Ups

- **Ingredients:** 1 small whole-grain tortilla, ¼ cup shredded cheese, ¼ cup diced vegetables (cucumbers, carrots)
- **Preparation:** Sprinkle cheese and veggies on the tortilla, roll up, and slice into bite-sized pieces.

14. Sweet Potato and Black Bean Tacos

- **Ingredients:** 1 small sweet potato (diced), ¼ cup black beans, 1 small whole-grain tortilla, 1 tbsp sour cream
- **Preparation:** Cook sweet potato until tender, place in tortilla with black beans and sour cream.

15. Pumpkin Pancakes

- **Ingredients:** ½ cup pumpkin puree, 1 egg, ¼ cup whole wheat flour, 1 tsp cinnamon
- **Preparation:** Mix all ingredients and cook small pancakes on a non-stick pan until golden.

16. Mini Pizza Bagels

- **Ingredients:** 2 mini whole-grain bagels, ¼ cup tomato sauce, ¼ cup shredded cheese, ¼ cup diced veggies (bell peppers, mushrooms)
- **Preparation:** Spread sauce on bagels, top with cheese and veggies, and bake at 350°F (175°C) for 10 minutes.

17. Broccoli and Cheese Quiche

- **Ingredients:** ½ cup chopped broccoli, ¼ cup shredded cheese, 2 eggs, ¼ cup milk
- **Preparation:** Mix all ingredients, pour into a greased pie dish, and bake at 350°F (175°C) for 25 minutes.

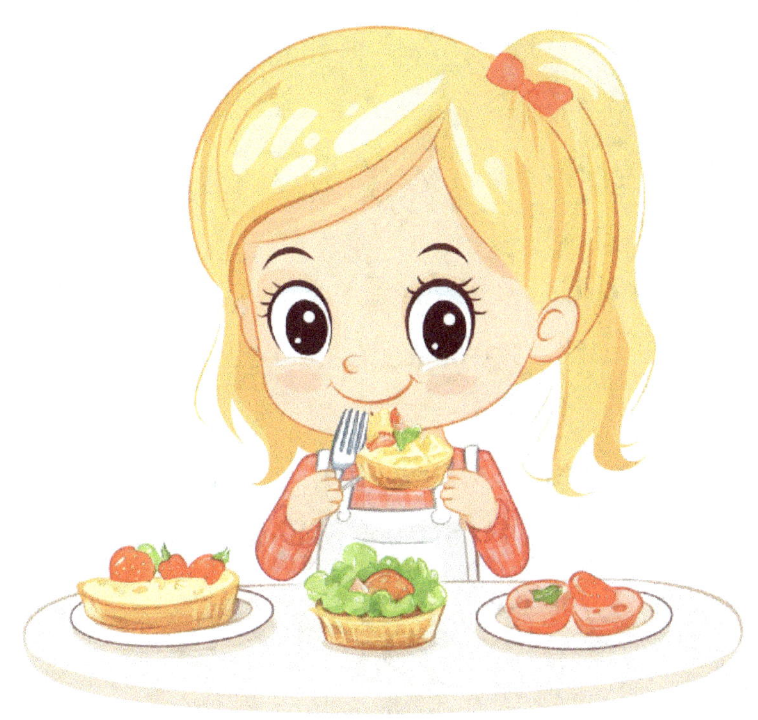

18. Baked Apple Slices with Cinnamon

- **Ingredients:** 1 apple (sliced), 1 tsp cinnamon, 1 tsp honey
- **Preparation:** Arrange apple slices on a baking sheet, sprinkle with cinnamon and honey, and bake at 350°F (175°C) for 15 minutes.

19. Turkey and Cheese Wrap

- **Ingredients:** 1 small whole-grain tortilla, 2 slices turkey breast, ¼ cup shredded cheese, 1 lettuce leaf
- **Preparation:** Place turkey, cheese, and lettuce on the tortilla, roll up, and slice into smaller pieces.

20. Cottage Cheese and Fruit Bowl

- **Ingredients:** ½ cup cottage cheese, ¼ cup diced fruit (peaches, berries), 1 tsp honey (optional)
- **Preparation:** Mix cottage cheese with fruit and drizzle with honey if desired.

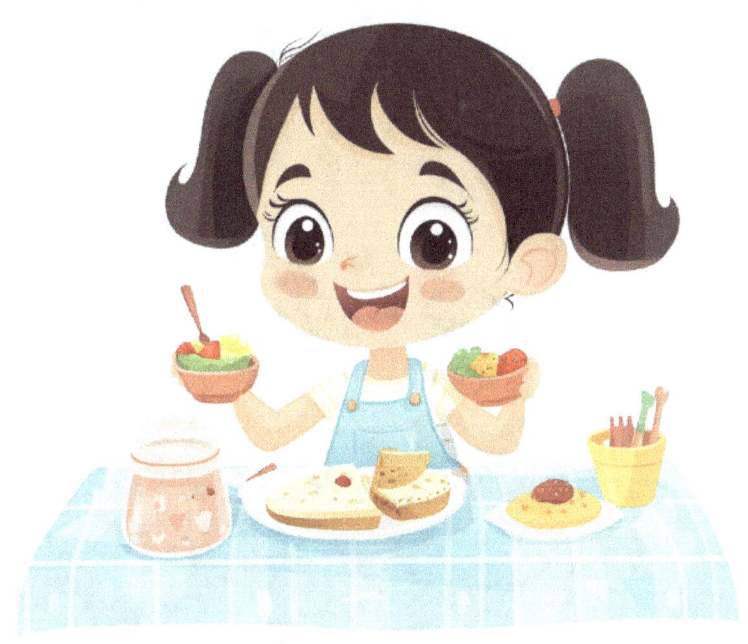

21. Zucchini Fritters

- **Ingredients:** 1 small zucchini (grated), 1 egg, ¼ cup whole wheat flour, salt to taste
- **Preparation:** Mix ingredients, form small fritters, and cook in a non-stick pan until golden brown.

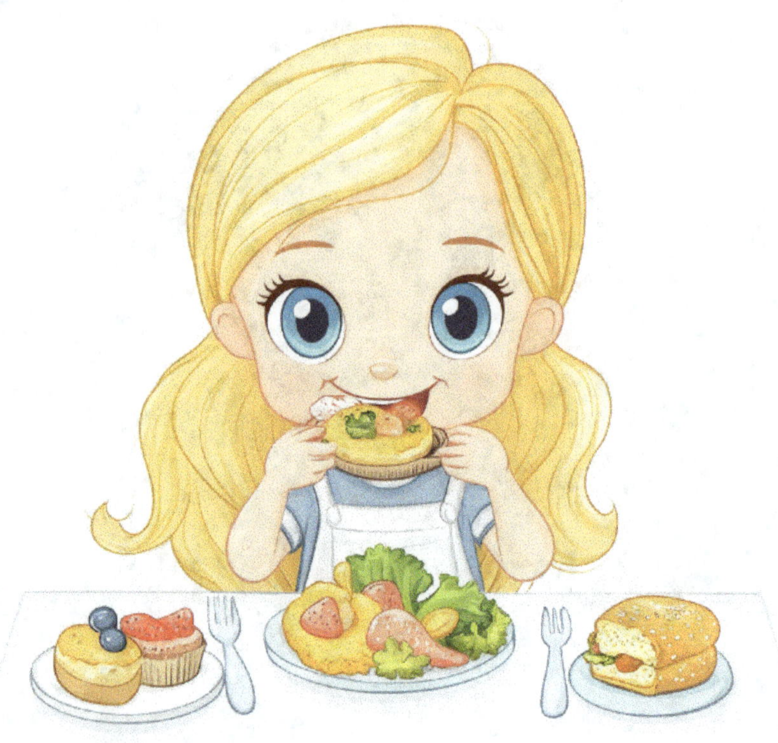

22. Carrot and Apple Muffins

- **Ingredients:** 1 cup whole wheat flour, 1 grated carrot, 1 grated apple, ¼ cup sugar, 1 egg, ¼ cup milk, 1 tsp baking powder
- **Preparation:** Mix all ingredients, pour into a muffin tin, and bake at 350°F (175°C) for 20 minutes.

23. Avocado and Banana Smoothie

- **Ingredients:** ½ avocado, 1 banana, ½ cup milk or yogurt, 1 tsp honey
- **Preparation:** Blend all ingredients until smooth.

24. Vegetable and Hummus Sandwich

- **Ingredients:** 1 slice whole-grain bread, 1 tbsp hummus, ¼ cup sliced veggies (cucumbers, bell peppers)
- **Preparation:** Spread hummus on bread, top with sliced veggies, and fold the bread in half.

25. Cheese and Tomato Omelette

- **Ingredients:** 2 eggs, ¼ cup diced tomatoes, ¼ cup shredded cheese, salt to taste
- **Preparation:** Whisk eggs, pour into a pan, add tomatoes and cheese, and cook until eggs are set.

26. Baked Banana with Cinnamon

- **Ingredients:** 1 banana (sliced), 1 tsp cinnamon, 1 tsp honey
- **Preparation:** Arrange banana slices on a baking sheet, sprinkle with cinnamon and honey, and bake at 350°F (175°C) for 10 minutes.

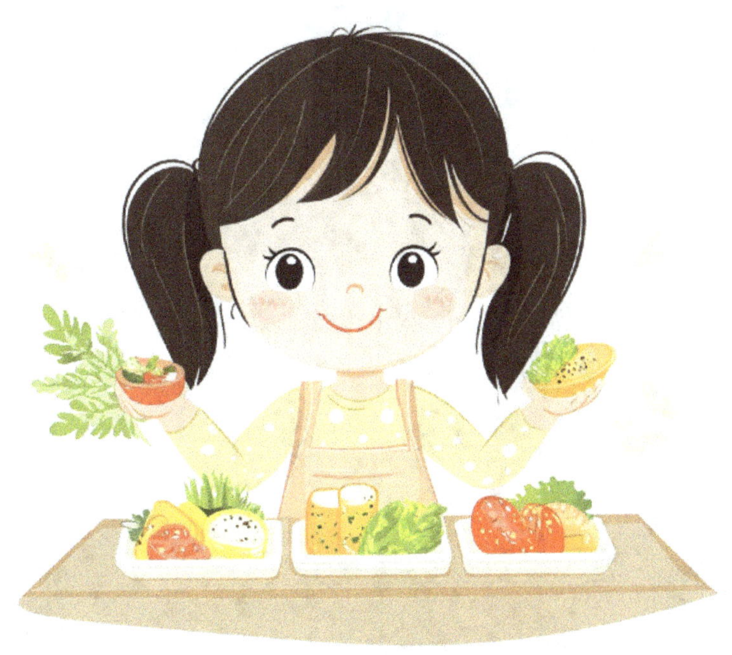

27. Spinach and Feta Quesadilla

- **Ingredients:** 1 small whole-grain tortilla, ¼ cup chopped spinach, ¼ cup crumbled feta cheese

- **Preparation:** Place spinach and feta on one half of the tortilla, fold, and cook in a pan until cheese melts.

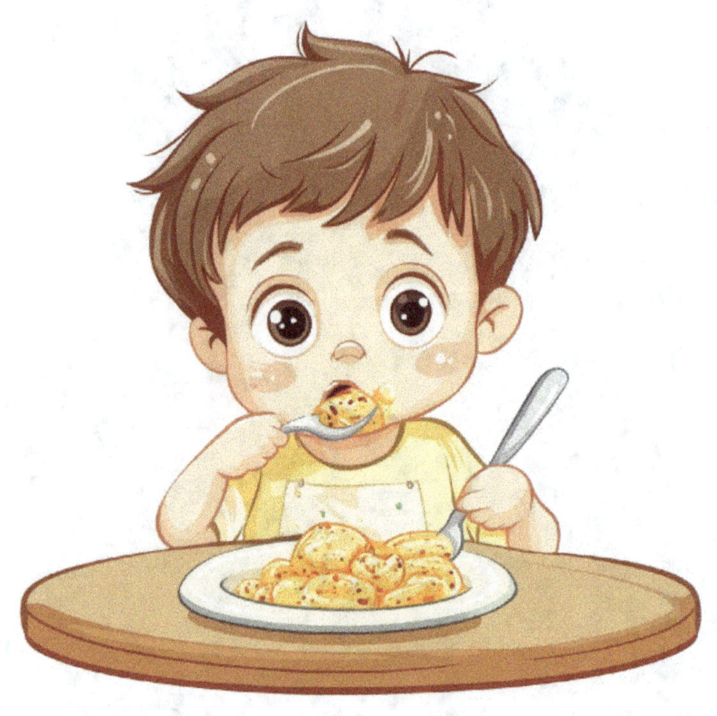

28. Sweet Potato Pancakes

- **Ingredients:** ½ cup mashed sweet potato, 1 egg, ¼ cup whole wheat flour, 1 tsp cinnamon
- **Preparation:** Mix all ingredients and cook small pancakes on a non-stick pan until golden.

29. Peanut Butter and Jelly Roll-Ups

- **Ingredients:** 1 small whole-grain tortilla, 1 tbsp peanut butter, 1 tbsp fruit preserves
- **Preparation:** Spread peanut butter and preserves on the tortilla, roll up, and slice into bite-sized pieces.

30. Egg Muffins with Veggies

- **Ingredients:** 2 eggs, ¼ cup diced bell peppers, ¼ cup spinach, salt to taste
- **Preparation:** Whisk eggs, mix in veggies, pour into a greased muffin tin, and bake at 350°F (175°C) for 15 minutes.

31. Fruit and Yogurt Popsicles

- **Ingredients:** 1 cup plain yogurt, ½ cup mixed berries, 1 tsp honey
- **Preparation:** Blend yogurt, berries, and honey, pour into popsicle molds, and freeze until solid.

32. Cheese and Apple Sandwich

- **Ingredients:** 1 slice whole-grain bread, 1 slice cheese, ½ apple (thinly sliced)
- **Preparation:** Place cheese and apple slices on bread, fold the bread in half, and toast if desired.

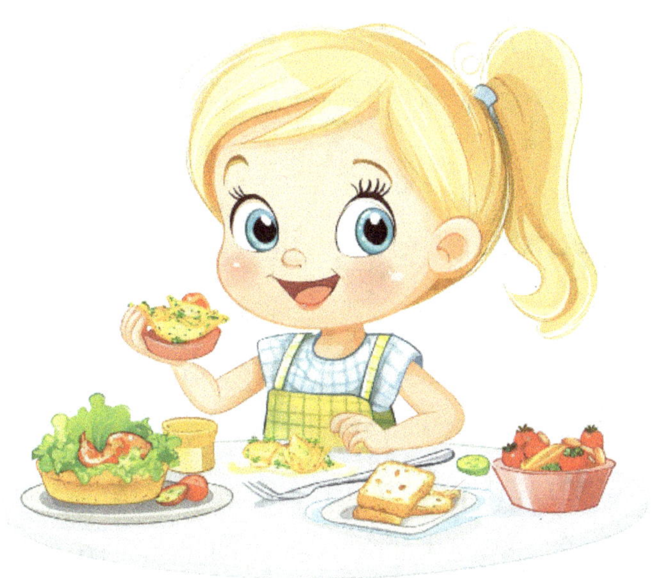

1. Baked Salmon with Sweet Potatoes

- **Ingredients:** 1 small salmon fillet, 1 small sweet potato, 1 tsp olive oil, pinch of salt
- **Preparation:** Preheat oven to 375°F (190°C). Slice sweet potato into rounds and toss with olive oil and salt. Place on a baking

sheet with salmon. Bake for 20 minutes or until salmon is cooked through.

2. Chicken and Vegetable Stir-Fry

- **Ingredients:** ½ cup diced chicken breast, ¼ cup broccoli florets, ¼ cup bell peppers, 1 tbsp soy sauce, 1 tsp olive oil
- **Preparation:** Heat olive oil in a pan, add chicken, and cook until browned. Add vegetables and soy sauce, stir-fry until tender.

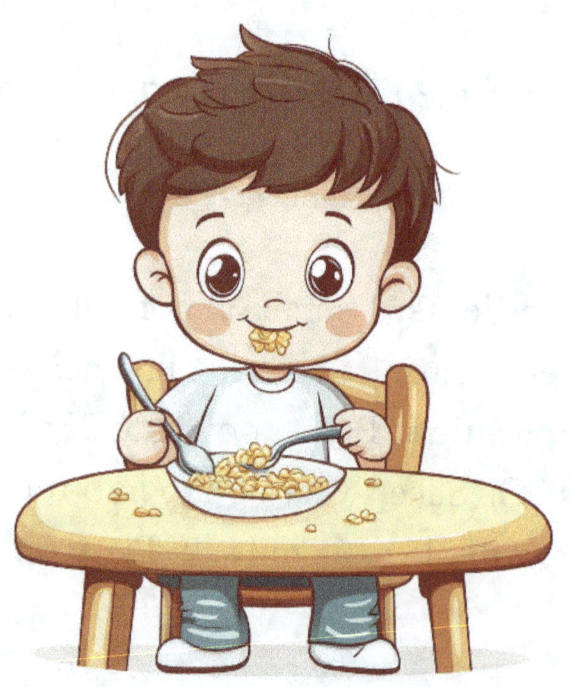

3. Turkey Meatballs with Mashed Potatoes

- **Ingredients:** ¼ lb ground turkey, ¼ cup breadcrumbs, 1 egg, 1 small potato, 1 tbsp butter, ¼ cup milk
- **Preparation:** Mix turkey, breadcrumbs, and egg, form small meatballs, and bake at 350°F (175°C) for 15 minutes. Boil and mash the potato with butter and milk.

4. Vegetable Soup

- **Ingredients:** ½ cup diced carrots, ½ cup diced potatoes, ¼ cup peas, 2 cups vegetable broth
- **Preparation:** Simmer vegetables in broth until tender. Puree for younger children if needed.

5. Baked Chicken Tenders

- **Ingredients:** ¼ lb chicken breast strips, ¼ cup breadcrumbs, 1 egg, 1 tbsp olive oil
- **Preparation:** Preheat oven to 375°F (190°C). Dip chicken in beaten egg, coat with breadcrumbs, and bake for 20 minutes until golden and cooked through.

6. Lentil Stew

- **Ingredients:** ½ cup lentils, ¼ cup diced carrots, ¼ cup diced celery, 2 cups vegetable broth
- **Preparation:** Simmer lentils and vegetables in broth until tender.

7. *Spaghetti with Tomato Sauce*

- **Ingredients:** ½ cup whole-grain spaghetti, ¼ cup tomato sauce, 1 tbsp grated Parmesan cheese

- **Preparation:** Cook spaghetti according to package instructions. Warm tomato sauce and mix with cooked spaghetti, then top with cheese.

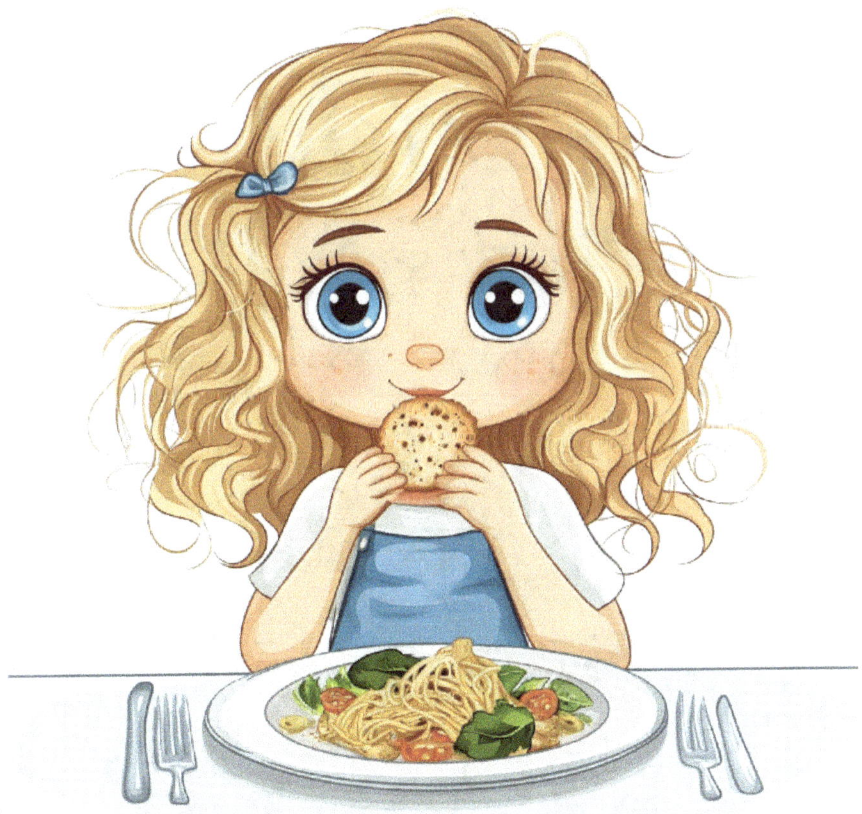

8. Vegetable and Cheese Quesadilla

- **Ingredients:** 1 small whole-grain tortilla, ¼ cup shredded cheese, ¼ cup diced vegetables (zucchini, bell peppers)
- **Preparation:** Place cheese and vegetables on one half of the tortilla, fold, and cook in a pan until cheese melts.

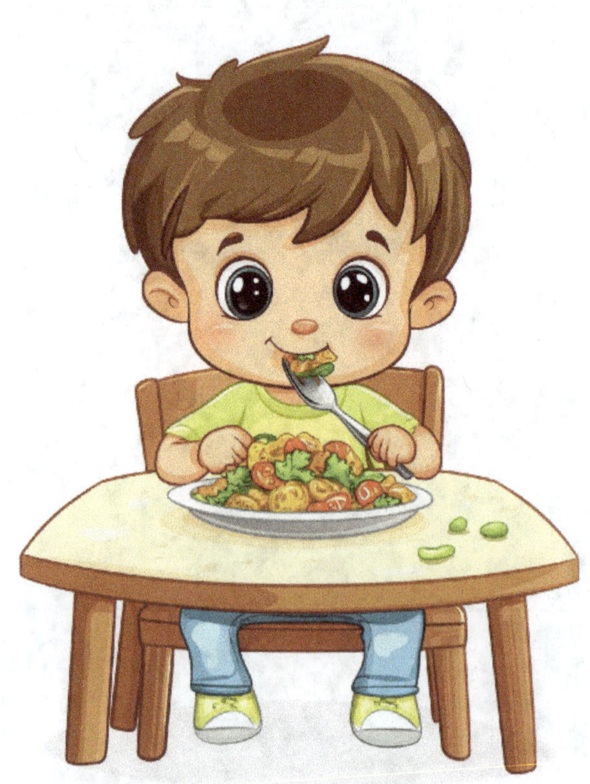

9. Chicken and Rice Casserole

- **Ingredients:** ½ cup cooked rice, ¼ cup diced chicken, ¼ cup mixed vegetables, 2 tbsp cream of chicken soup
- **Preparation:** Mix all ingredients, pour into a baking dish, and bake at 350°F (175°C) for 20 minutes.

10. Fish Sticks with Green Beans

- **Ingredients:** 2-3 fish sticks, ¼ cup steamed green beans, 1 tbsp olive oil
- **Preparation:** Bake fish sticks according to package instructions. Steam green beans and toss with olive oil.

11. Vegetable Risotto

- **Ingredients:** ½ cup Arborio rice, ¼ cup diced zucchini, ¼ cup diced carrots, 2 cups vegetable broth
- **Preparation:** Cook rice in broth, stirring frequently. Add vegetables halfway through cooking.

12. Baked Zucchini Boats

- **Ingredients:** 1 small zucchini, ¼ cup tomato sauce, ¼ cup shredded cheese
- **Preparation:** Slice zucchini in half lengthwise, scoop out the center, fill with tomato sauce and cheese, and bake at 375°F (190°C) for 15 minutes.

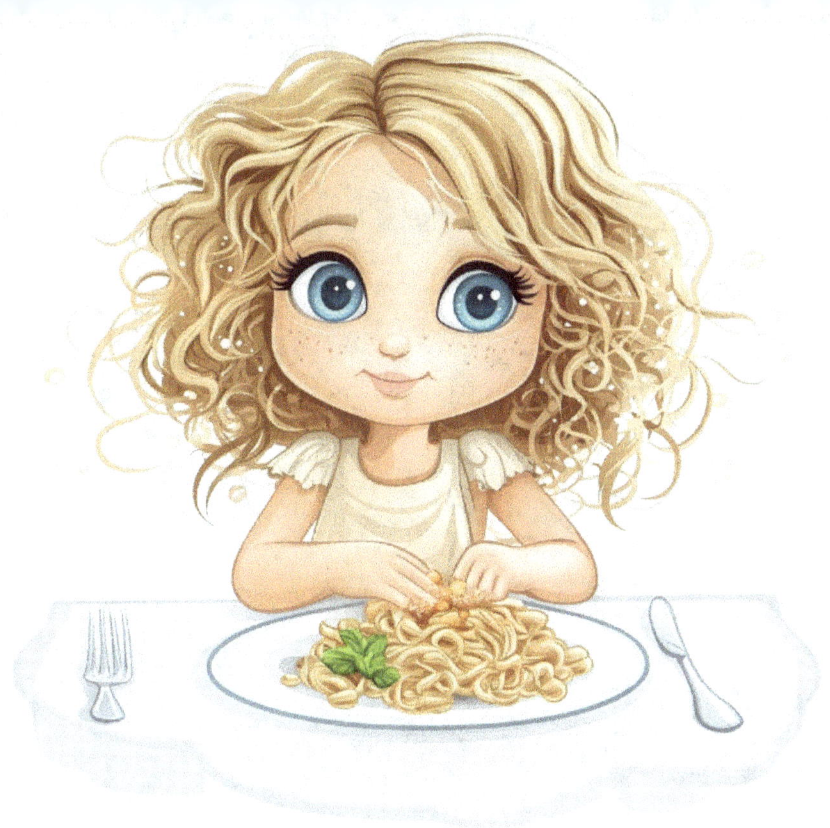

13. Turkey and Spinach Lasagna

- **Ingredients:** ¼ lb ground turkey, ½ cup spinach, ½ cup ricotta cheese, ¼ cup shredded mozzarella, 2 lasagna noodles, ¼ cup tomato sauce
- **Preparation:** Layer cooked lasagna noodles with turkey, spinach, ricotta, and sauce. Top with mozzarella and bake at 350°F (175°C) for 20 minutes.

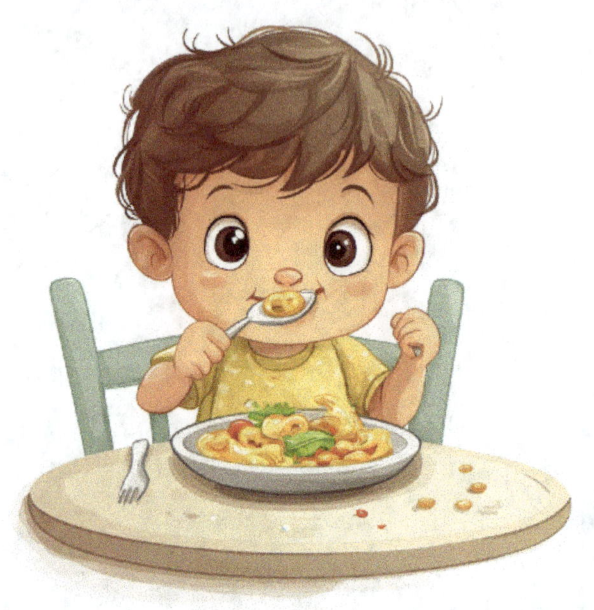

14. Vegetable Fried Rice

- **Ingredients:** ½ cup cooked rice, ¼ cup diced carrots, ¼ cup peas, 1 egg, 1 tbsp soy sauce

- **Preparation:** Scramble the egg in a pan, add rice and vegetables, and stir-fry with soy sauce.

15. Baked Chicken with Quinoa

- **Ingredients:** ¼ lb chicken breast, ½ cup cooked quinoa, ¼ cup steamed broccoli
- **Preparation:** Season chicken with salt and pepper, bake at 375°F (190°C) for 20 minutes, and serve with quinoa and broccoli.

16. Cheesy Broccoli and Rice

- **Ingredients:** ½ cup cooked rice, ¼ cup steamed broccoli, ¼ cup shredded cheese
- **Preparation:** Mix rice with broccoli and cheese, and bakc at 350°F (175°C) for 10 minutes until cheese is melted.

17. Turkey and Avocado Wrap

- **Ingredients:** 1 small whole-grain tortilla, 2 slices turkey breast, ¼ avocado (sliced)
- **Preparation:** Place turkey and avocado on the tortilla, roll up, and slice into smaller pieces.

18. Sweet Potato and Black Bean Tacos

- **Ingredients:** 1 small sweet potato (diced), ¼ cup black beans, 1 small whole-grain tortilla, 1 tbsp sour cream
- **Preparation:** Cook sweet potato until tender, place in tortilla with black beans and sour cream.

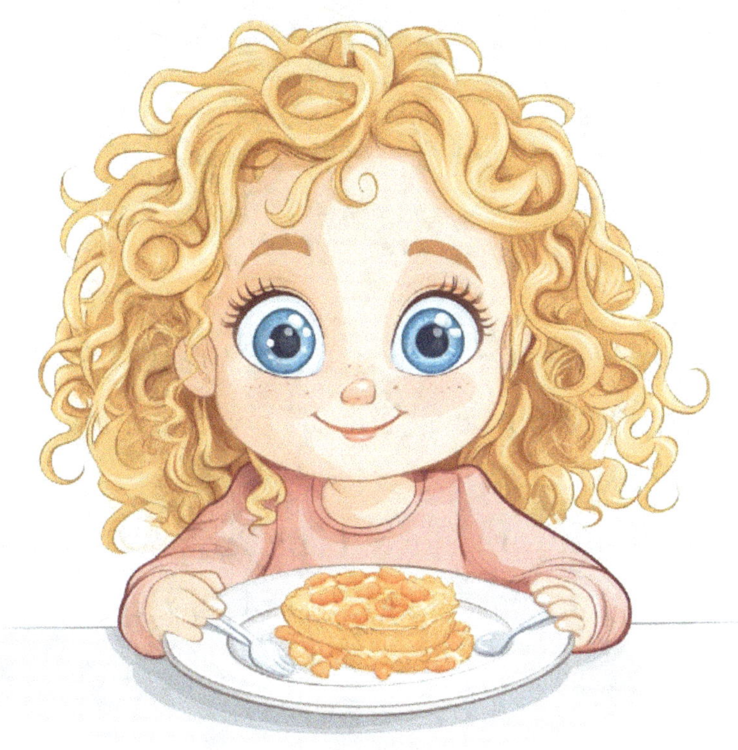

19. Mini Turkey Meatloaf

- **Ingredients:** ¼ lb ground turkey, ¼ cup breadcrumbs, 1 egg, ¼ cup ketchup
- **Preparation:** Mix turkey, breadcrumbs, and egg, shape into mini loaves, top with ketchup, and bake at 350°F (175°C) for 20 minutes.

20. Chicken and Vegetable Kabobs

- **Ingredients:** ¼ lb chicken breast (cubed), ¼ cup bell peppers (cubed), ¼ cup zucchini (cubed)
- **Preparation:** Thread chicken and vegetables onto skewers and grill until cooked through.

21. Macaroni and Cheese with Peas

- **Ingredients:** ½ cup whole-grain macaroni, ¼ cup shredded cheese, ¼ cup frozen peas, 1 tbsp butter
- **Preparation:** Cook macaroni and peas together, drain, and stir in butter and cheese until melted.

22. Baked Cod with Carrots

- **Ingredients:** 1 small cod fillet, ¼ cup diced carrots, 1 tsp olive oil, pinch of salt
- **Preparation:** Preheat oven to 375°F (190°C). Toss carrots with olive oil and salt, place on a baking sheet with cod, and bake for 20 minutes.

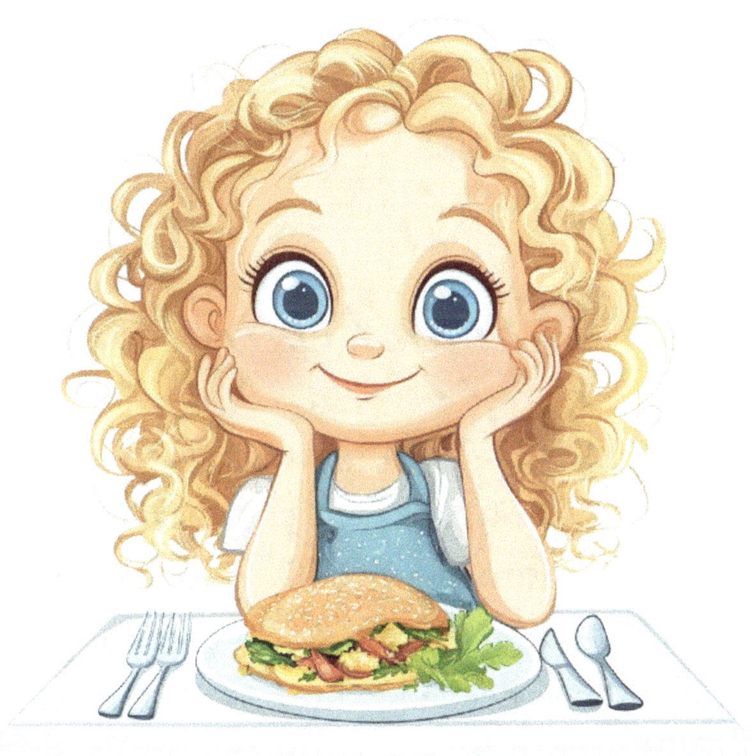

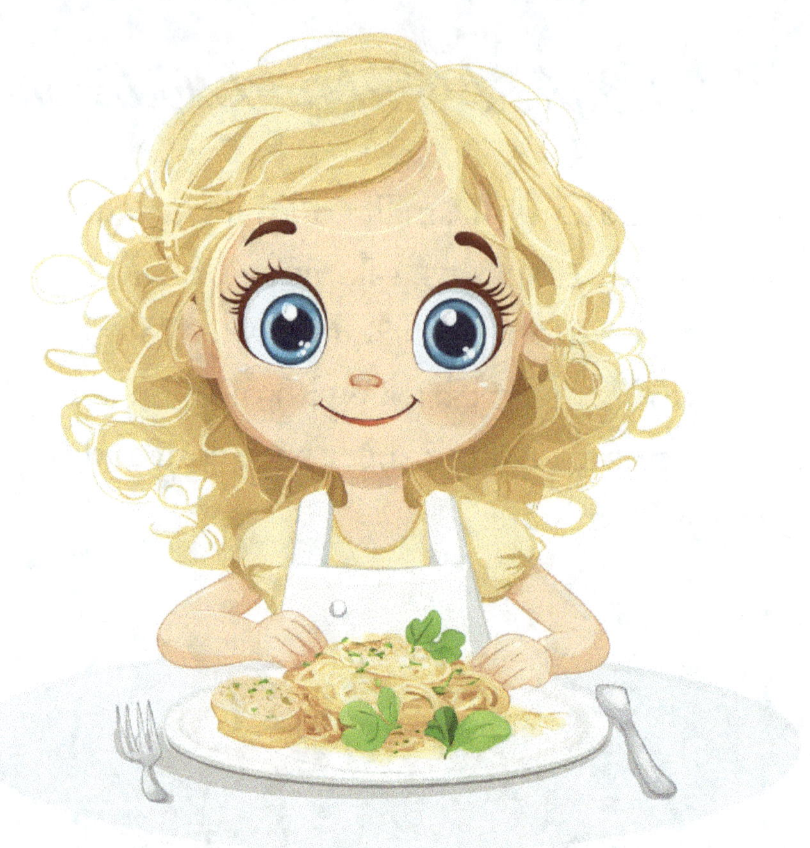

23. Lentil and Carrot Soup

- **Ingredients:** ½ cup lentils, 2 carrots (sliced), 1 small onion (diced), 2 cups vegetable broth
- **Preparation:** Simmer all ingredients until lentils and carrots are soft. Puree for younger children if needed.

24. Chicken and Avocado Salad

- **Ingredients:** ½ cup diced chicken, ¼ avocado (sliced), 1 tbsp olive oil, 1 tsp lemon juice
- **Preparation:** Mix chicken and avocado with olive oil and lemon juice.

25. Vegetable and Cheese Frittata

- **Ingredients:** 2 eggs, ¼ cup diced vegetables (zucchini, bell peppers), ¼ cup shredded cheese
- **Preparation:** Whisk eggs, add vegetables and cheese, and bake at 350°F (175°C) for 15 minutes.

26. Baked Chicken and Butternut Squash

- **Ingredients:** ¼ lb chicken breast, ½ cup diced butternut squash, 1 tsp olive oil
- **Preparation:** Toss squash with olive oil, place on a baking sheet with chicken, and bake at 375°F (190°C) for 25 minutes.

27. Turkey and Vegetable Skewers

- **Ingredients:** ¼ lb ground turkey (formed into small balls), ¼ cup bell peppers, ¼ cup zucchini
- **Preparation:** Thread turkey and vegetables onto skewers and grill or bake until cooked through.

28. Cheesy Cauliflower Bake

- **Ingredients:** ½ cup steamed cauliflower, ¼ cup shredded cheese, 1 tbsp breadcrumbs
- **Preparation:** Preheat oven to 350°F (175°C). Mix cauliflower with cheese, top with breadcrumbs, and bake for 15 minutes.

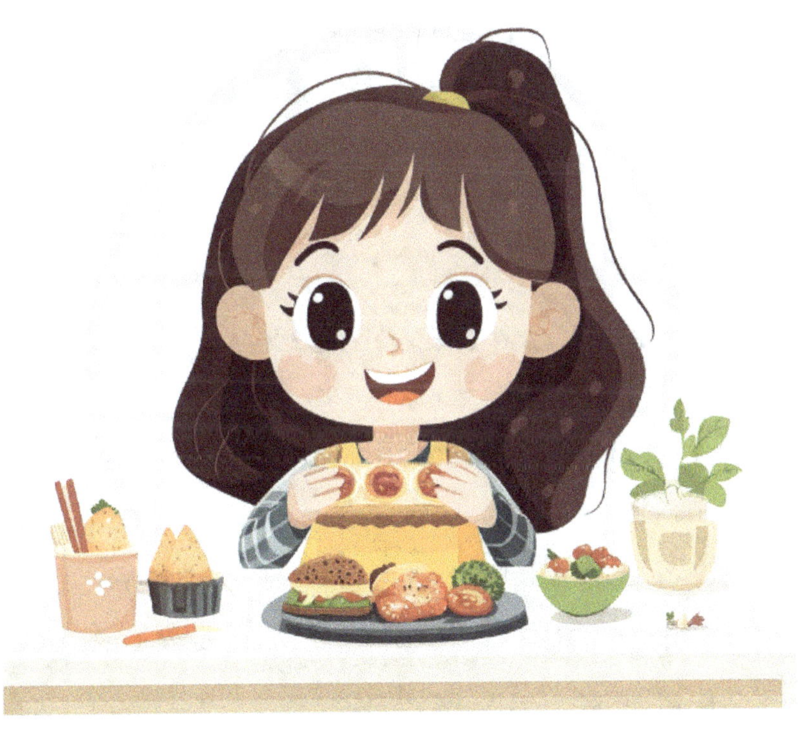

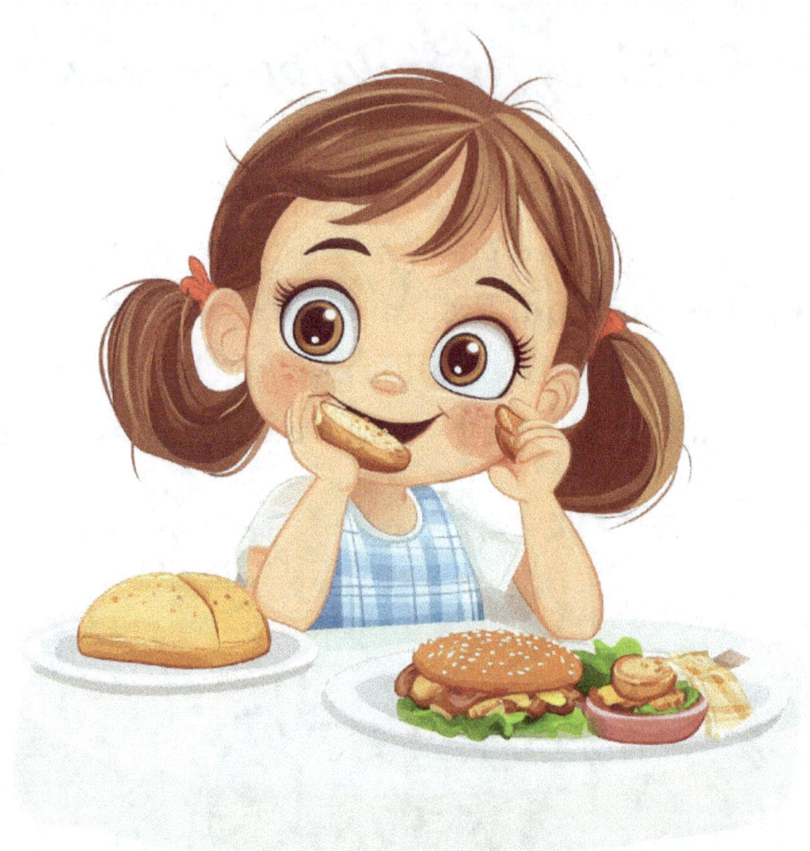

29. Chicken and Bean Burrito

- **Ingredients:** 1 small whole-grain tortilla, ¼ cup diced chicken, ¼ cup black beans, 2 tbsp shredded cheese
- **Preparation:** Fill tortilla with chicken, beans, and cheese, then roll up.

30. Vegetable and Chicken Soup

- **Ingredients:** ½ cup diced chicken, ¼ cup diced carrots, ¼ cup diced potatoes, 2 cups chicken broth
- **Preparation:** Simmer chicken and vegetables in broth until tender.

31. Baked Eggplant Parmesan

- **Ingredients:** ½ small eggplant (sliced), ¼ cup tomato sauce, ¼ cup shredded mozzarella, 1 tbsp breadcrumbs
- **Preparation:** Preheat oven to 375°F (190°C). Layer eggplant slices with tomato sauce and cheese in a baking dish, sprinkle with breadcrumbs, and bake for 20 minutes.

32. Stuffed Bell Peppers

- **Ingredients:** 1 small bell pepper (halved and seeded), ¼ cup cooked quinoa, ¼ cup diced chicken, ¼ cup tomato sauce
- **Preparation:** Mix quinoa, chicken, and tomato sauce. Stuff into bell pepper halves and bake at 350°F (175°C) for 25 minutes.

33. Vegetable and Chicken Stir-Fry

- **Ingredients:** ½ cup diced chicken, ¼ cup broccoli florets, ¼ cup sliced carrots, 1 tbsp soy sauce, 1 tsp olive oil
- **Preparation:** Heat olive oil in a pan, add chicken and cook until browned. Add vegetables and soy sauce, stir-fry until tender.

34. Baked Potato with Broccoli and Cheese

- **Ingredients:** 1 small potato, ¼ cup steamed broccoli, ¼ cup shredded cheese
- **Preparation:** Bake potato at 375°F (190°C) for 45 minutes. Top with steamed broccoli and cheese, then return to oven until cheese is melted.

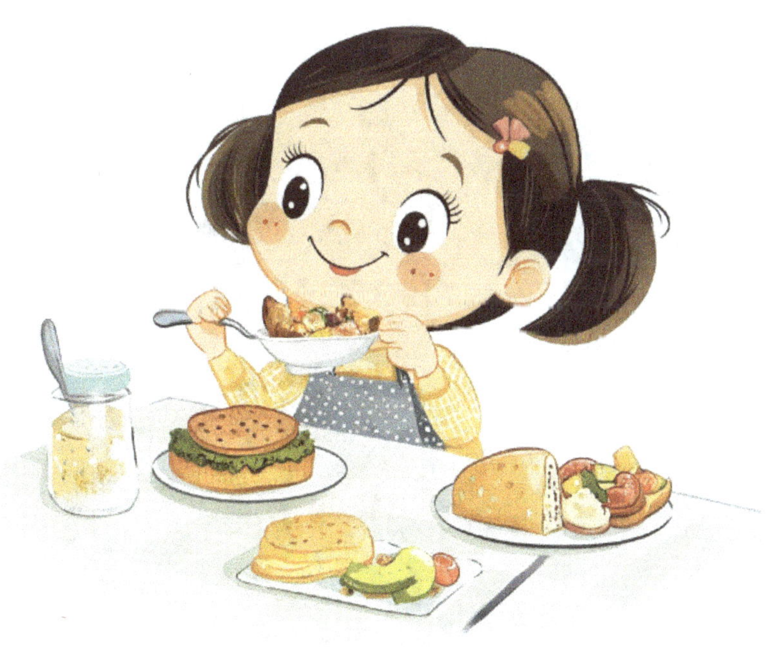

35. Turkey and Spinach Stuffed Shells

- **Ingredients:** 4 large pasta shells, ¼ cup cooked ground turkey, ¼ cup ricotta cheese, ¼ cup spinach, ¼ cup tomato sauce
- **Preparation:** Mix turkey, ricotta, and spinach. Stuff into cooked pasta shells, place in a baking dish, cover with tomato sauce, and bake at 350°F (175°C) for 20 minutes.

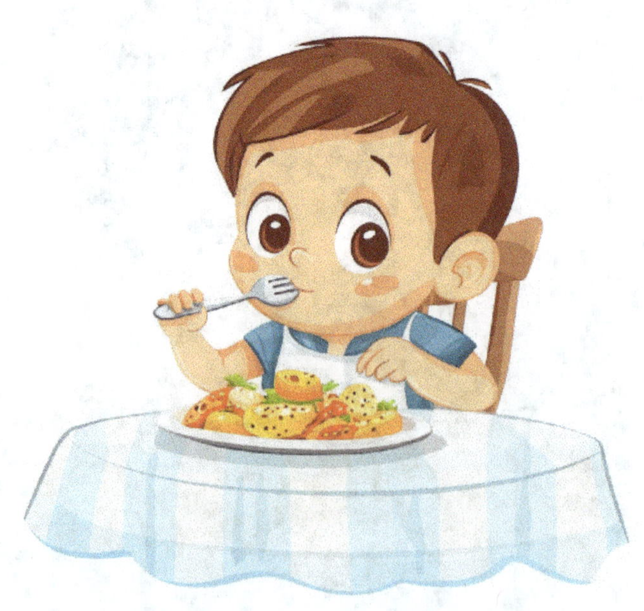

36. Grilled Chicken and Zucchini

- **Ingredients:** ¼ lb chicken breast, ¼ cup zucchini (sliced), 1 tsp olive oil, salt to taste
- **Preparation:** Marinate chicken in olive oil and salt, then grill with zucchini slices until cooked through.

37. Cheesy Cauliflower Mac and Cheese

- **Ingredients:** ½ cup whole-grain macaroni, ¼ cup steamed cauliflower, ¼ cup shredded cheese, 1 tbsp butter
- **Preparation:** Cook macaroni, drain, and mix with cauliflower, cheese, and butter until melted.

38. Salmon Patties

- **Ingredients:** ¼ cup cooked salmon (flaked), ¼ cup breadcrumbs, 1 egg, 1 tsp lemon juice
- **Preparation:** Mix ingredients, form into small patties, and cook in a pan until golden on both sides.

39. Chicken and Corn Chowder

- **Ingredients:** ½ cup diced chicken, ¼ cup corn kernels, ¼ cup diced potatoes, 2 cups chicken broth
- **Preparation:** Simmer chicken, corn, and potatoes in broth until tender.

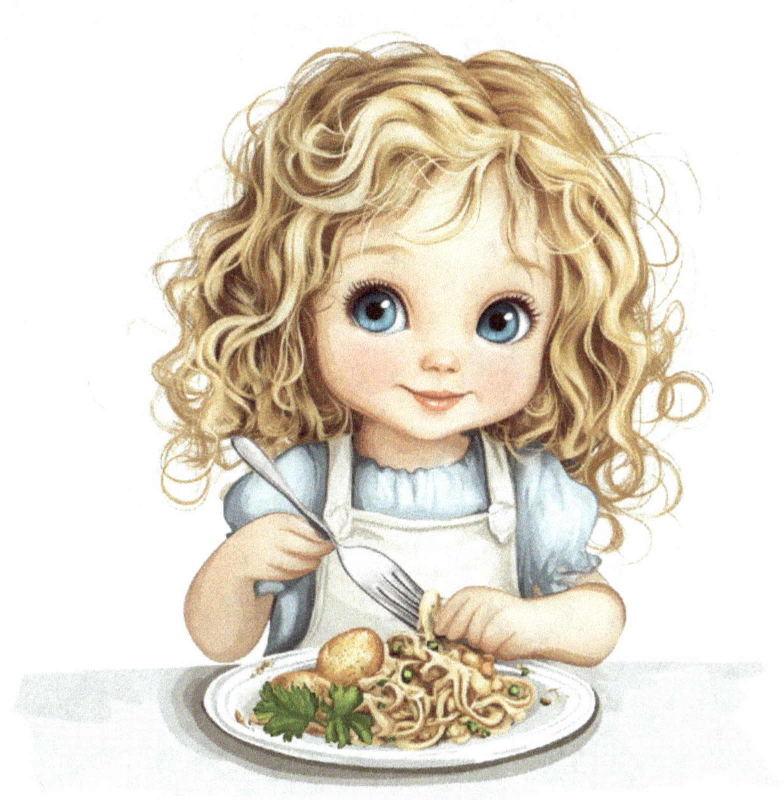

40. Baked Tilapia with Sweet Potato Fries

- **Ingredients:** 1 small tilapia fillet, 1 small sweet potato (cut into fries), 1 tsp olive oil, salt to taste
- **Preparation:** Toss sweet potato fries with olive oil and salt, bake at 375°F (190°C) for 25 minutes. Bake tilapia for 15 minutes or until cooked through.

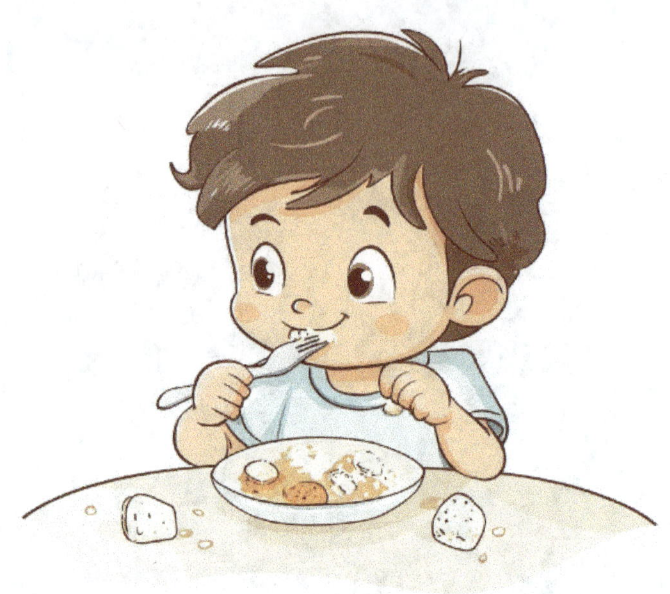

41. Spinach and Cheese Stuffed Chicken

- **Ingredients:** ¼ lb chicken breast (butterflied), ¼ cup spinach, ¼ cup shredded cheese
- **Preparation:** Stuff chicken breast with spinach and cheese, secure with toothpicks, and bake at 375°F (190°C) for 25 minutes.

42. Vegetable and Chicken Curry

- **Ingredients:** ½ cup diced chicken, ¼ cup diced carrots, ¼ cup diced potatoes, 1 tbsp curry powder, 1 cup coconut milk
- **Preparation:** Cook chicken in a pan, add vegetables, curry powder, and coconut milk. Simmer until vegetables are tender.

43. Vegetable and Lentil Tacos

- **Ingredients:** ¼ cup cooked lentils, ¼ cup diced tomatoes, ¼ cup shredded lettuce, 1 small whole-grain tortilla, 1 tbsp sour cream
- **Preparation:** Fill tortilla with lentils, tomatoes, lettuce, and sour cream, then roll up.

44. Chicken and Apple Sausage with Mashed Sweet Potatoes

- **Ingredients:** 1 chicken and apple sausage, 1 small sweet potato, 1 tbsp butter, ¼ cup milk
- **Preparation:** Boil sweet potato and mash with butter and milk. Cook sausage according to package instructions and serve with mashed sweet potatoes.

45. Shrimp and Vegetable Stir-Fry

- **Ingredients:** ¼ cup shrimp (peeled), ¼ cup broccoli florets, ¼ cup bell peppers (sliced), 1 tbsp soy sauce, 1 tsp olive oil
- **Preparation:** Heat olive oil in a pan, add shrimp, and cook until pink. Add vegetables and soy sauce, stir-fry until tender.

46. Vegetable and Cheese Calzone

- **Ingredients:** ¼ cup shredded mozzarella, ¼ cup diced bell peppers, ¼ cup spinach, 1 small whole-grain pizza dough
- **Preparation:** Roll out dough, fill with cheese and vegetables, fold over, seal edges, and bake at 375°F (190°C) for 15 minutes.

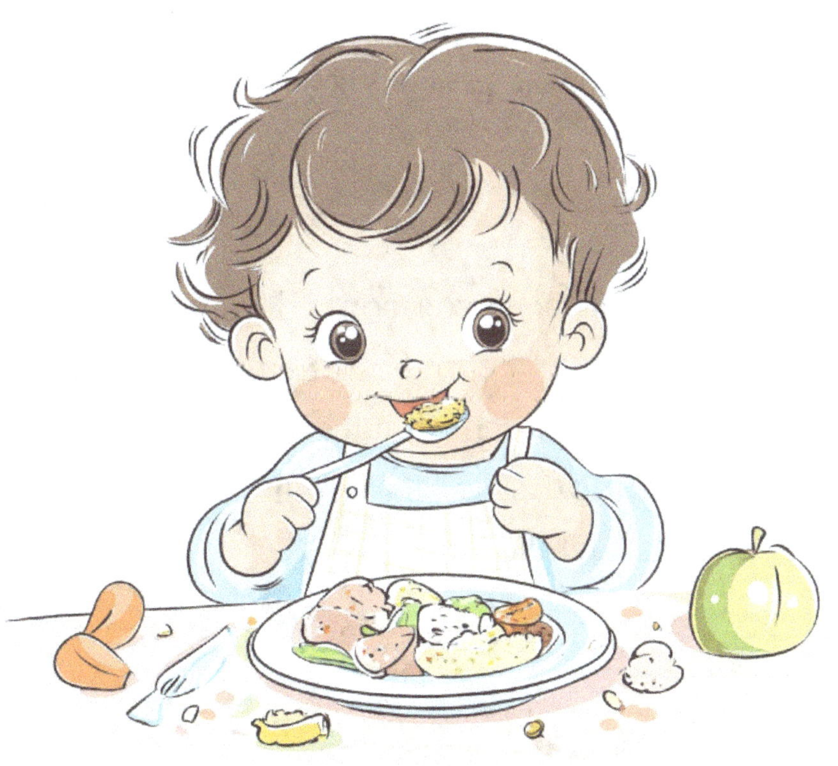

47. Chicken and Rice Soup

- **Ingredients:** ½ cup diced chicken, ¼ cup cooked rice, ¼ cup diced carrots, 2 cups chicken broth
- **Preparation:** Simmer chicken, rice, and carrots in broth until tender.

48. Quinoa and Black Bean Salad

- **Ingredients:** ½ cup cooked quinoa, ¼ cup black beans, ¼ cup diced tomatoes, 1 tbsp olive oil, 1 tsp lemon juice
- **Preparation:** Mix all ingredients together and serve chilled.

49. Baked Turkey and Sweet Potato Nuggets

- **Ingredients:** ¼ lb ground turkey, ¼ cup mashed sweet potato, ¼ cup breadcrumbs, 1 egg
- **Preparation:** Mix ingredients, form into nuggets, and bake at 375°F (190°C) for 15 minutes.

50. Vegetable and Cheese Stuffed Mushrooms

- **Ingredients:** 4 large mushrooms (stems removed), ¼ cup diced vegetables (spinach, bell peppers), ¼ cup shredded cheese
- **Preparation:** Stuff mushrooms with vegetables and cheese, bake at 375°F (190°C) for 15 minutes.

healthy dessert recipes for children, with minimal or no added sugar

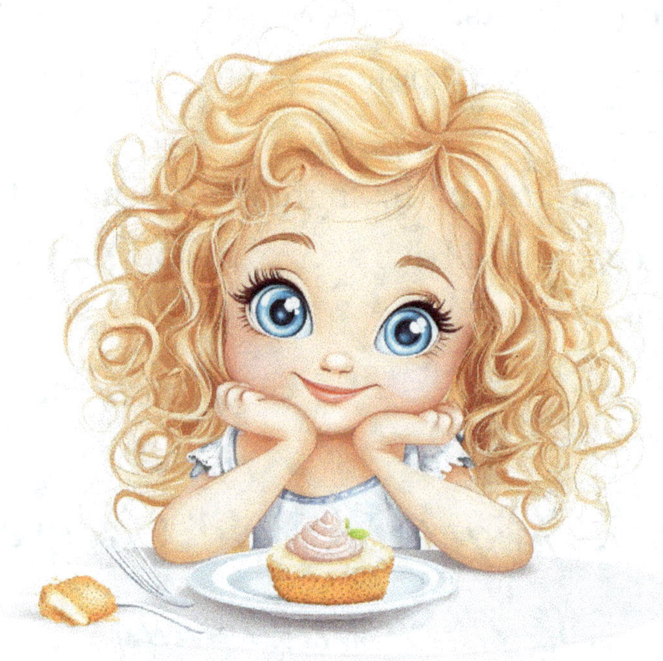

1. Apple Slices with Peanut Butter

- **Ingredients:** 1 apple (sliced), 2 tbsp natural peanut butter
- **Preparation:** Spread peanut butter on apple slices and serve.

2. Greek Yogurt with Berries

- **Ingredients:** ½ cup plain Greek yogurt, ¼ cup mixed berries (strawberries, blueberries, raspberries)
- **Preparation:** Mix berries into yogurt and serve chilled.

3. Banana Oat Cookies

- **Ingredients:** 2 ripe bananas, 1 cup oats, ¼ cup raisins
- **Preparation:** Preheat oven to 350°F (175°C). Mash bananas and mix with oats and raisins. Drop spoonfuls onto a baking sheet and bake for 12-15 minutes.

4. Chia Seed Pudding

- **Ingredients:** 2 tbsp chia seeds, ½ cup almond milk, 1 tsp honey (optional)
- **Preparation:** Mix chia seeds with almond milk and refrigerate for 2 hours until it thickens. Add honey for sweetness if desired.

5. Baked Cinnamon Apples

- **Ingredients:** 2 apples (sliced), 1 tsp cinnamon
- **Preparation:** Preheat oven to 375°F (190°C). Toss apple slices with cinnamon and bake for 20 minutes.

6. Frozen Yogurt Bark

- **Ingredients:** 1 cup Greek yogurt, ¼ cup mixed berries, 1 tbsp honey (optional)
- **Preparation:** Spread yogurt on a baking sheet lined with parchment paper. Top with berries and freeze for 2 hours. Break into pieces and serve.

7. Avocado Chocolate Mousse

- **Ingredients:** 1 ripe avocado, 2 tbsp cocoa powder, 1 tbsp honey (optional)
- **Preparation:** Blend avocado, cocoa powder, and honey until smooth. Serve chilled.

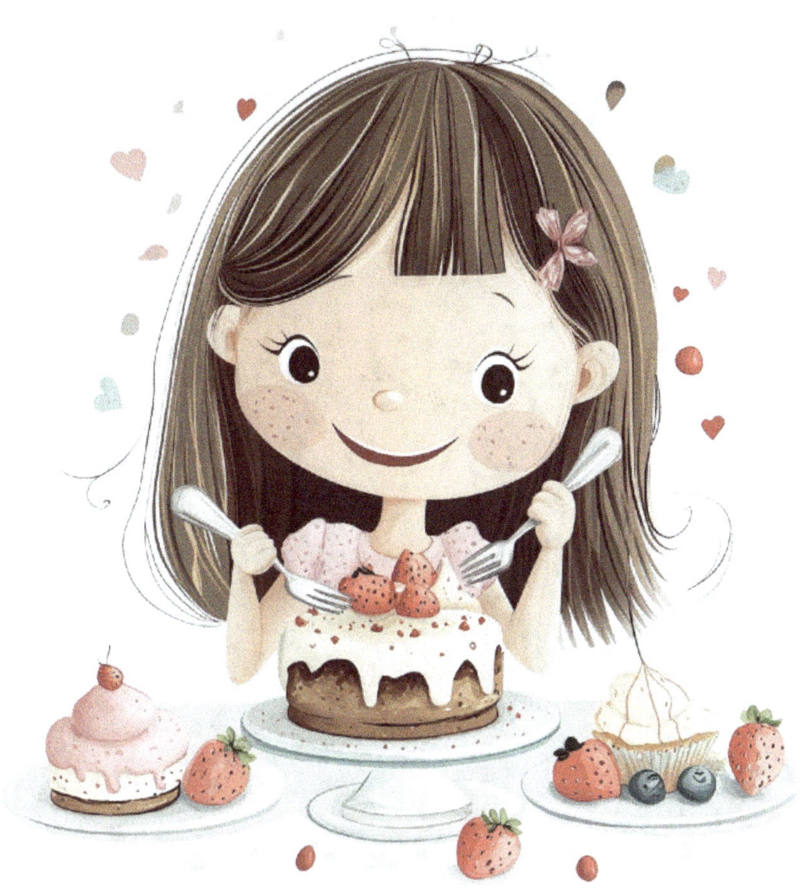

8. Coconut Date Balls

- **Ingredients:** 1 cup pitted dates, ½ cup shredded coconut
- **Preparation:** Blend dates until smooth. Roll into small balls and coat with shredded coconut.

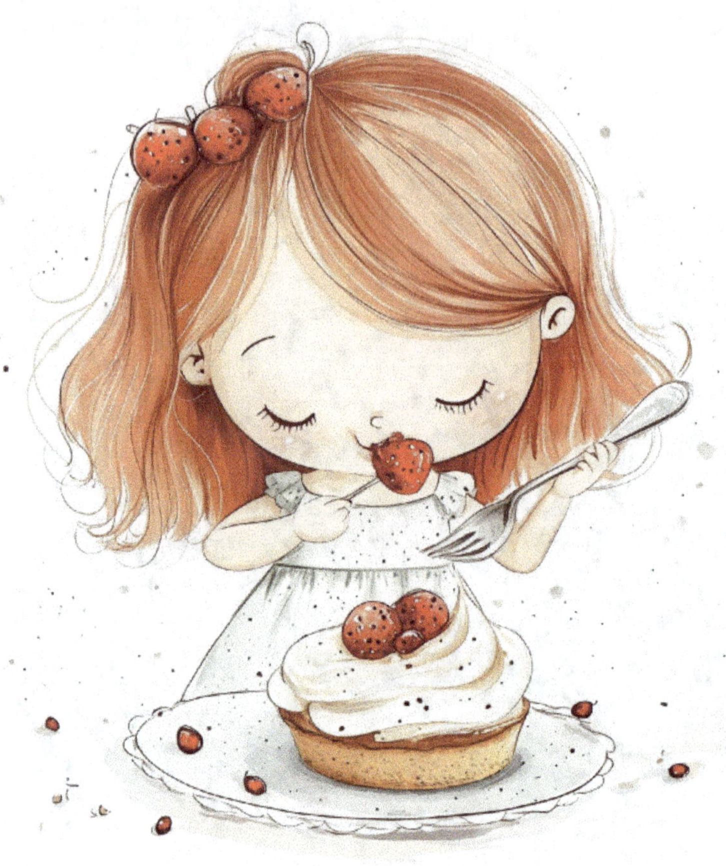

9. Banana Ice Cream

- **Ingredients:** 2 ripe bananas
- **Preparation:** Slice bananas and freeze. Blend frozen slices until creamy, and serve immediately.

10. Carrot Cake Bites

- **Ingredients:** 1 cup shredded carrots, 1 cup oats, ½ cup dates, ½ tsp cinnamon
- **Preparation:** Blend all ingredients, form into small balls, and refrigerate for 1 hour.

11. Apple and Oat Bars

- **Ingredients:** 1 cup oats, 2 apples (grated), 1 tsp cinnamon
- **Preparation:** Mix oats, grated apples, and cinnamon. Press into a baking dish and bake at 350°F (175°C) for 20 minutes.

12. Frozen Banana Pops

- **Ingredients:** 2 bananas, ¼ cup Greek yogurt, 2 tbsp crushed nuts
- **Preparation:** Dip banana halves in yogurt, roll in crushed nuts, and freeze for 2 hours.

13. Mango Sorbet

- **Ingredients:** 1 ripe mango, 1 tbsp lime juice
- **Preparation:** Blend mango and lime juice until smooth, then freeze for 2 hours before serving.

14. Pumpkin Oat Muffins

- **Ingredients:** 1 cup oats, ½ cup pumpkin puree, 1 tsp cinnamon, 1 egg
- **Preparation:** Mix all ingredients, spoon into a muffin tin, and bake at 350°F (175°C) for 15-20 minutes.

15. Blueberry Coconut Energy Bites

- **Ingredients:** 1 cup oats, ¼ cup dried blueberries, ¼ cup shredded coconut, 2 tbsp honey
- **Preparation:** Mix all ingredients, form into balls, and refrigerate for 1 hour.

16. Baked Pears with Almonds

- **Ingredients:** 2 pears (halved), 2 tbsp chopped almonds, 1 tsp cinnamon
- **Preparation:** Preheat oven to 350°F (175°C). Place pear halves in a baking dish, sprinkle with almonds and cinnamon, and bake for 20 minutes.

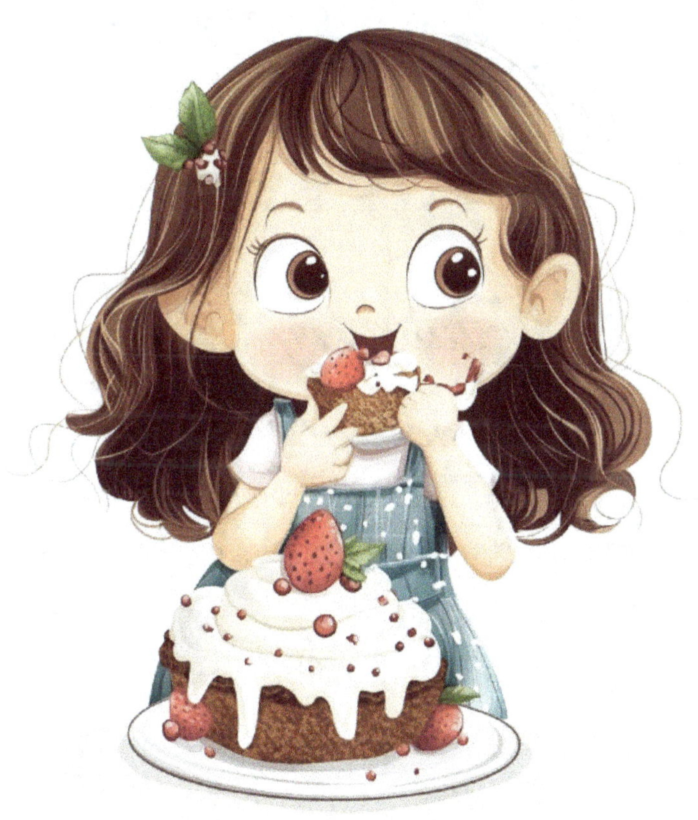

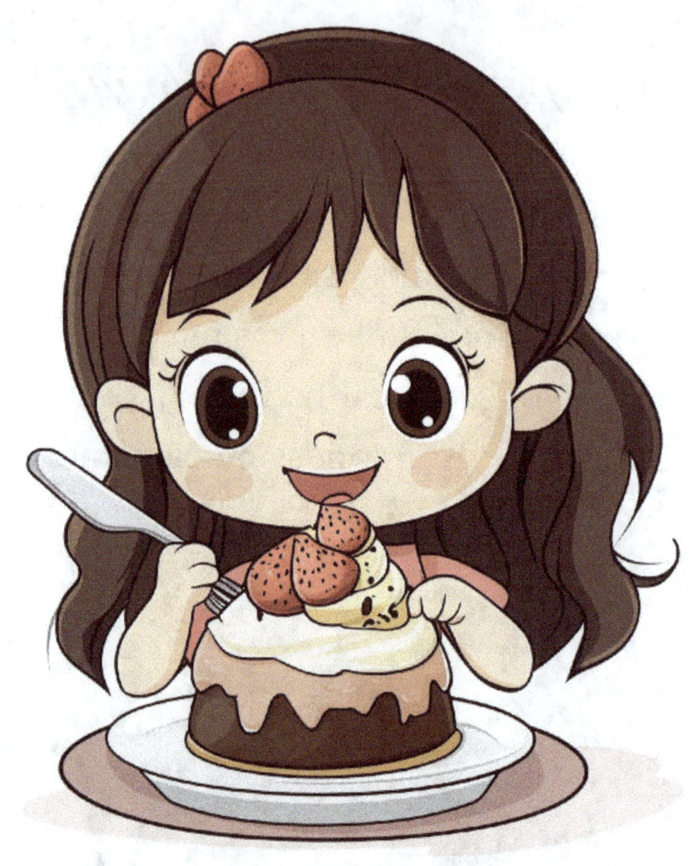

17. Strawberry Banana Smoothie

- **Ingredients:** 1 banana, ½ cup strawberries, ½ cup Greek yogurt
- **Preparation:** Blend all ingredients until smooth and serve immediately.

18. Oatmeal Raisin Cookies

- **Ingredients:** 1 cup oats, 1 ripe banana, ¼ cup raisins, 1 tsp cinnamon
- **Preparation:** Preheat oven to 350°F (175°C). Mash banana and mix with oats, raisins, and cinnamon. Drop spoonfuls onto a baking sheet and bake for 12-15 minutes.

19. Coconut Rice Pudding

- **Ingredients:** ½ cup cooked rice, ½ cup coconut milk, 1 tsp vanilla extract
- **Preparation:** Mix all ingredients in a saucepan and cook on low heat until thickened.

20. Apple and Cinnamon Rice Cakes

- **Ingredients:** 1 rice cake, ½ apple (sliced), 1 tsp cinnamon
- **Preparation:** Top rice cake with apple slices and sprinkle with cinnamon.

21. Zucchini Chocolate Muffins

- **Ingredients:** 1 cup grated zucchini, 1 egg, ¼ cup cocoa powder, ½ cup oats
- **Preparation:** Mix all ingredients, spoon into a muffin tin, and bake at 350°F (175°C) for 15-20 minutes.

22. Peach and Yogurt Parfait

- **Ingredients:** 1 peach (sliced), ½ cup Greek yogurt, 1 tbsp granola
- **Preparation:** Layer peach slices, yogurt, and granola in a glass and serve.

23. Homemade Applesauce

- **Ingredients:** 4 apples (peeled and chopped), 1 tsp cinnamon, ½ cup water
- **Preparation:** Simmer apples with water and cinnamon until soft, then mash or blend until smooth.

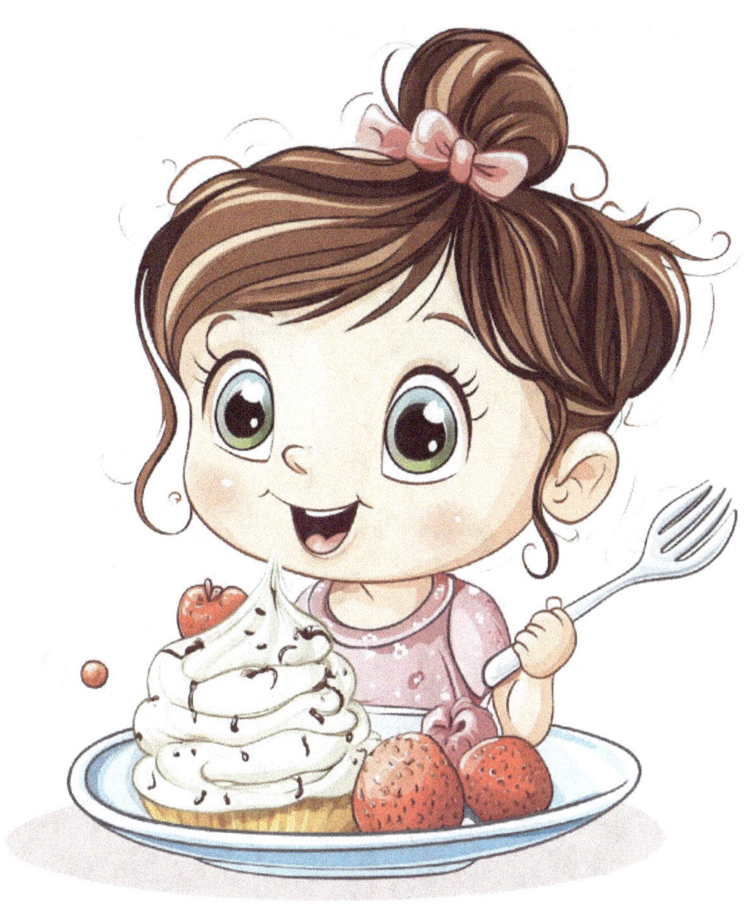

24. Berry Chia Jam

- **Ingredients:** 1 cup mixed berries, 2 tbsp chia seeds, 1 tbsp honey (optional)
- **Preparation:** Cook berries on low heat until they break down. Stir in chia seeds and honey, then refrigerate until thickened.

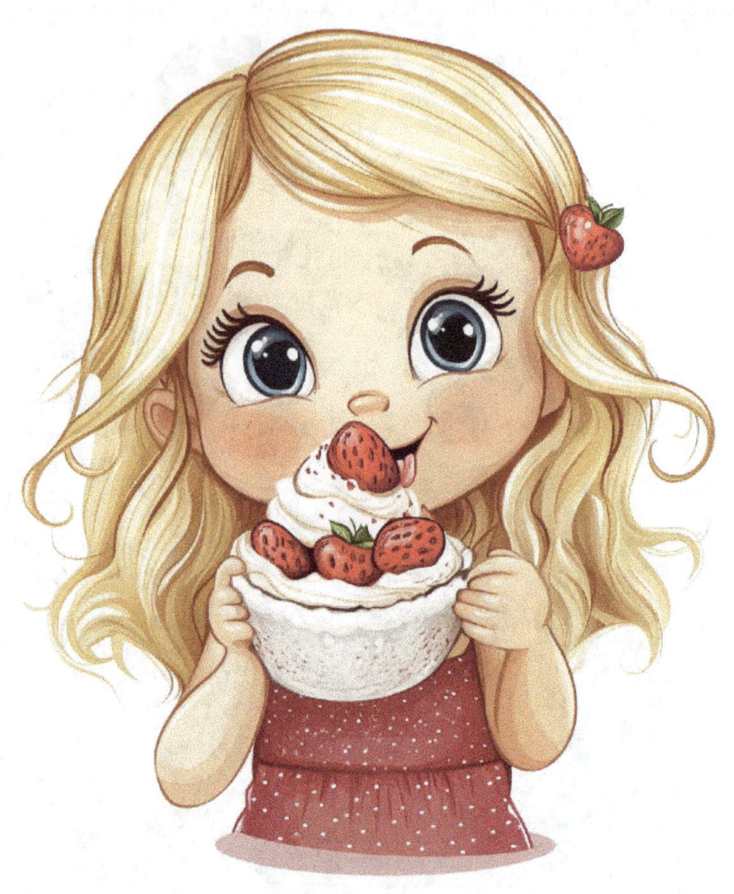

25. Sweet Potato Brownies

- **Ingredients:** 1 cup mashed sweet potato, ¼ cup cocoa powder, 1 egg
- **Preparation:** Mix all ingredients, spread in a baking dish, and bake at 350°F (175°C) for 20 minutes.

26. Frozen Yogurt Dots

- **Ingredients:** ½ cup Greek yogurt, 1 tbsp honey (optional)
- **Preparation:** Spoon small dots of yogurt onto a baking sheet and freeze for 2 hours.

27. Coconut Banana Bread

- **Ingredients:** 2 ripe bananas, 1 cup oats, ¼ cup shredded coconut, 1 egg
- **Preparation:** Mash bananas and mix with oats, coconut, and egg. Pour into a loaf pan and bake at 350°F (175°C) for 30 minutes.

28. Pumpkin Spice Energy Balls

- **Ingredients:** 1 cup oats, ½ cup pumpkin puree, 1 tsp pumpkin spice, 2 tbsp honey
- **Preparation:** Mix all ingredients, form into balls, and refrigerate for 1 hour.

29. Apple Cinnamon Chips

- **Ingredients:** 2 apples (thinly sliced), 1 tsp cinnamon
- **Preparation:** Preheat oven to 250°F (120°C). Place apple slices on a baking sheet, sprinkle with cinnamon, and bake for 1-2 hours until crisp.

30. Peanut Butter Banana Bites

- **Ingredients:** 1 banana, 2 tbsp natural peanut butter, ¼ cup crushed nuts
- **Preparation:** Slice banana, spread peanut butter between slices to make sandwiches, and roll in crushed nuts.

31. Frozen Yogurt-Covered Blueberries

- **Ingredients:** 1 cup blueberries, ½ cup Greek yogurt
- **Preparation:** Dip blueberries in Greek yogurt and place on a baking sheet. Freeze for 1-2 hours until firm.

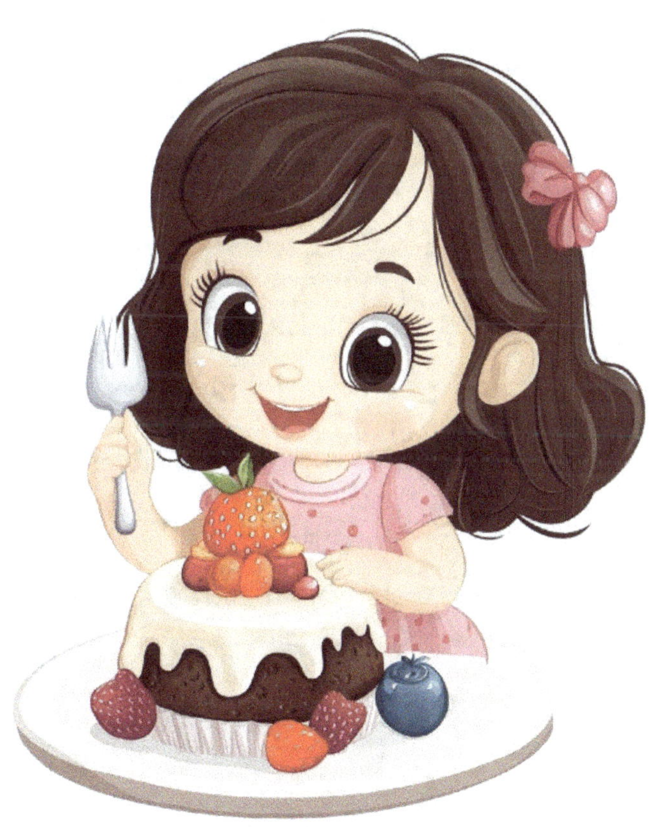

32. Carrot and Apple Muffins

- **Ingredients:** 1 cup grated carrots, 1 apple (grated), 1 cup oats, 1 egg
- **Preparation:** Mix all ingredients, spoon into a muffin tin, and bake at 350°F (175°C) for 20 minutes.

-

33. Baked Peaches with Greek Yogurt

- **Ingredients:** 2 peaches (halved), 1 cup Greek yogurt, 1 tsp cinnamon
- **Preparation:** Bake peach halves at 350°F (175°C) for 20 minutes. Serve with a dollop of Greek yogurt and a sprinkle of cinnamon.

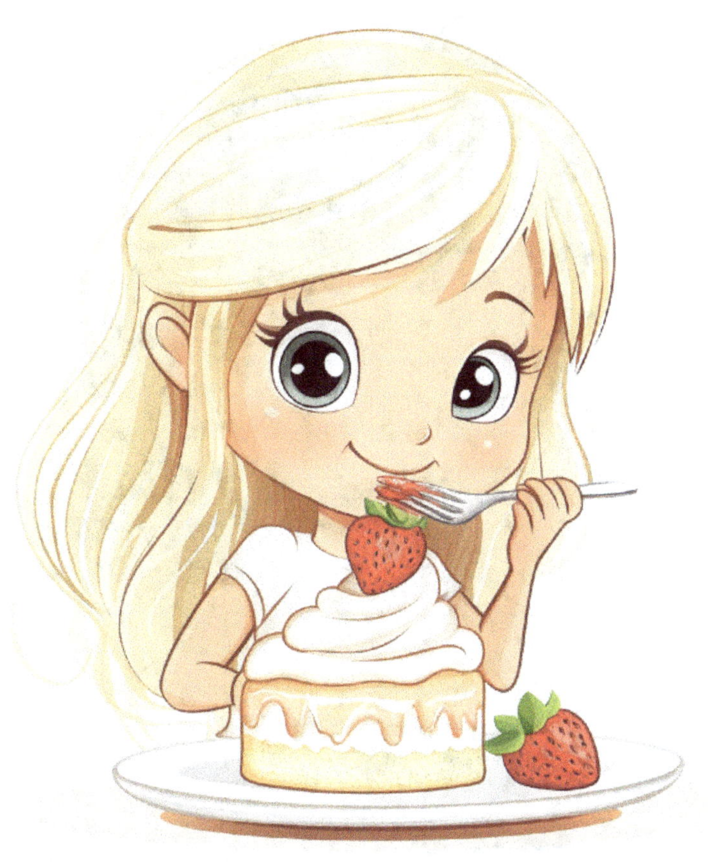

34. Avocado and Banana Pudding

- **Ingredients:** 1 ripe avocado, 1 ripe banana, 1 tsp vanilla extract
- **Preparation:** Blend avocado, banana, and vanilla extract until smooth. Serve chilled.

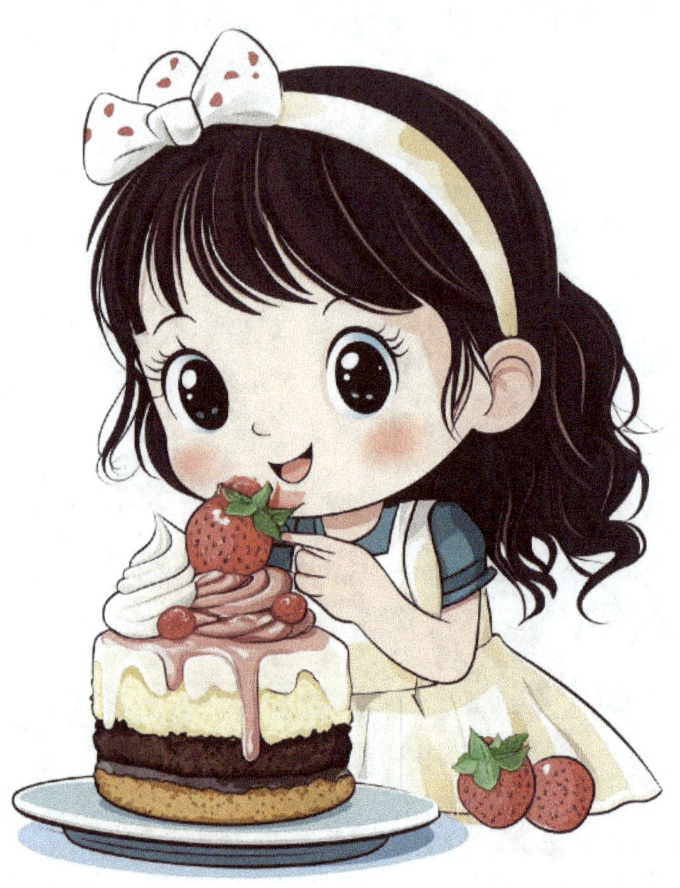

35. No-Bake Almond Butter Balls

- **Ingredients:** ½ cup almond butter, 1 cup oats, 2 tbsp honey (optional)
- **Preparation:** Mix all ingredients, form into balls, and refrigerate for 1 hour.

36. Pumpkin Yogurt Popsicles

- **Ingredients:** 1 cup pumpkin puree, 1 cup Greek yogurt, 1 tsp cinnamon
- **Preparation:** Mix all ingredients, pour into popsicle molds, and freeze for 4 hours.

37. Apple and Cheddar Quesadilla

- **Ingredients:** 1 small whole-grain tortilla, ½ apple (thinly sliced), ¼ cup shredded cheddar cheese
- **Preparation:** Place apple slices and cheese on half of the tortilla, fold, and cook in a skillet until cheese is melted.

38. Zucchini Bread

- **Ingredients:** 1 cup grated zucchini, 1 cup oats, 1 egg, 1 tsp cinnamon
- **Preparation:** Mix all ingredients, pour into a loaf pan, and bake at 350°F (175°C) for 30 minutes.

39. Sweet Potato and Apple Mash

- **Ingredients:** 1 small sweet potato (cooked and mashed), 1 apple (cooked and mashed), 1 tsp cinnamon
- **Preparation:** Mix mashed sweet potato, apple, and cinnamon together and serve warm.

40. Fruit and Nut Butter Sandwich

- **Ingredients:** 1 small whole-grain pita, 1 tbsp almond butter, ¼ cup sliced strawberries
- **Preparation:** Spread almond butter on the pita, top with sliced strawberries, and fold in half.

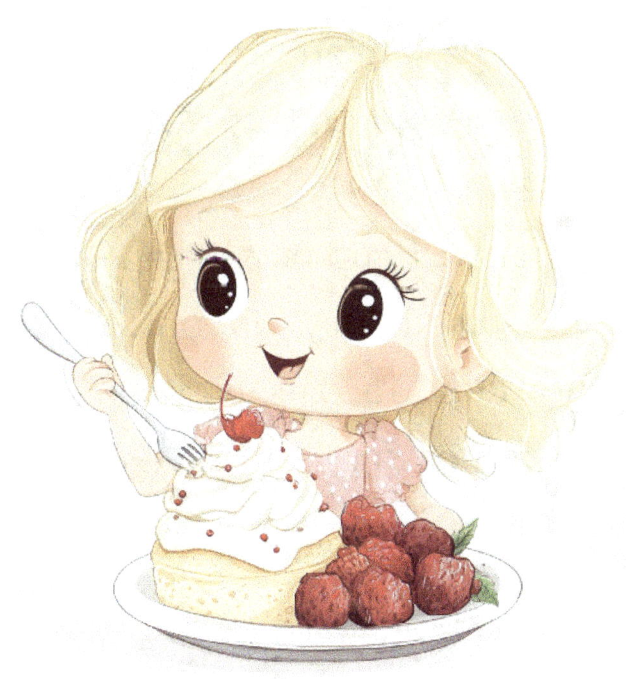

41. Baked Banana Chips

- **Ingredients:** 2 ripe bananas (thinly sliced)
- **Preparation:** Preheat oven to 200°F (95°C). Place banana slices on a baking sheet and bake for 1-2 hours until crisp.

42. Coconut Banana Bites

- **Ingredients:** 1 banana (sliced), ¼ cup shredded coconut
- **Preparation:** Roll banana slices in shredded coconut and freeze for 1 hour.

43. Berry Oat Bars

- **Ingredients:** 1 cup oats, 1 cup mixed berries, 2 tbsp honey (optional)
- **Preparation:** Mix oats, berries, and honey. Press into a baking dish and bake at 350°F (175°C) for 20 minutes.

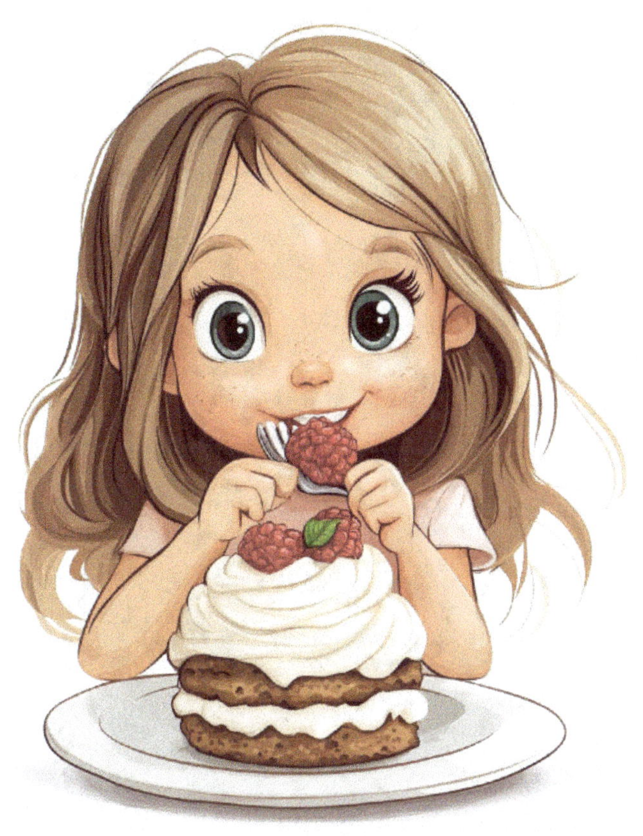

44. Cinnamon Baked Pears

- **Ingredients:** 2 pears (halved), 1 tsp cinnamon, 1 tbsp almond butter
- **Preparation:** Sprinkle pear halves with cinnamon and bake at 350°F (175°C) for 20 minutes. Drizzle with almond butter before serving.

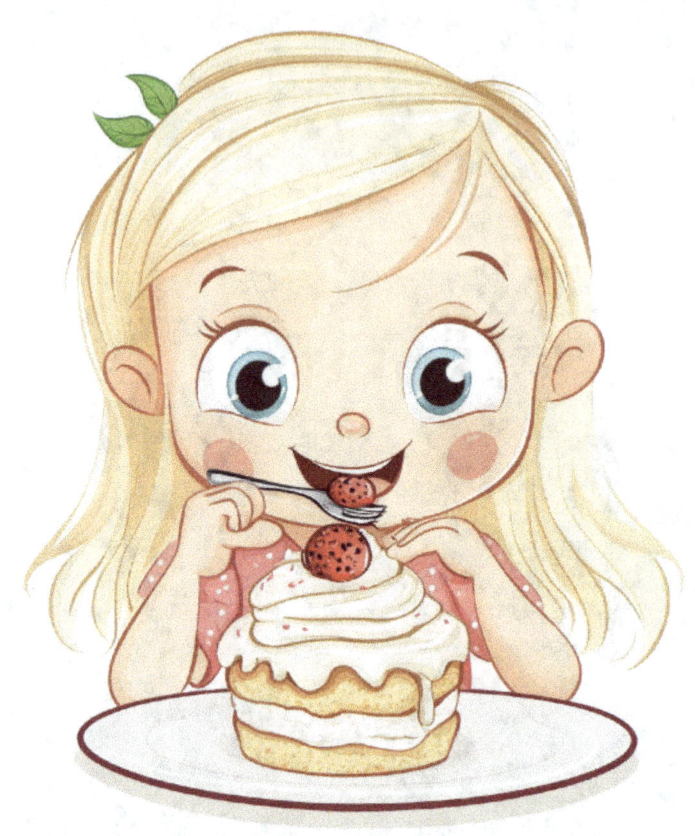

45. Watermelon Popsicles

- **Ingredients:** 2 cups watermelon (seeded and cubed)
- **Preparation:** Puree watermelon, pour into popsicle molds, and freeze for 4 hours.

46. Oatmeal Bites with Dried Fruit

- **Ingredients:** 1 cup oats, ¼ cup dried apricots (chopped), ¼ cup raisins, 2 tbsp honey (optional)
- **Preparation:** Mix all ingredients, form into balls, and refrigerate for 1 hour.

47. Baked Avocado Fries

- **Ingredients:** 1 avocado (sliced), ¼ cup breadcrumbs
- **Preparation:** Preheat oven to 375°F (190°C). Dip avocado slices in breadcrumbs and bake for 15 minutes.

48. Strawberry Chia Pudding

- **Ingredients:** 1 cup strawberries (pureed), 2 tbsp chia seeds, ½ cup almond milk
- **Preparation:** Mix pureed strawberries, chia seeds, and almond milk. Refrigerate for 2 hours until thickened.

49. Apple Cinnamon Roll-Ups

- **Ingredients:** 1 small whole-grain tortilla, ½ apple (thinly sliced), 1 tsp cinnamon
- **Preparation:** Place apple slices on the tortilla, sprinkle with cinnamon, roll up, and serve.

50. Homemade Applesauce Popsicles

- **Ingredients:** 1 cup unsweetened applesauce, 1 tsp cinnamon
- **Preparation:** Mix applesauce and cinnamon, pour into popsicle molds, and freeze for 4 hours.

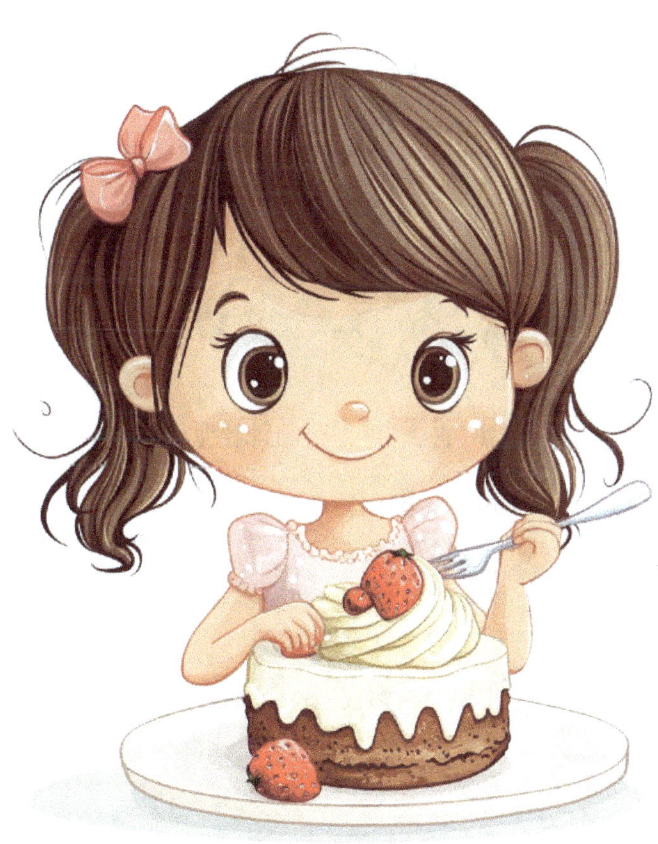

Dear Readers,

I want to express my heartfelt thanks for choosing this book and trusting me with the care of your little ones' nutrition. I hope it becomes a helpful and enjoyable companion on your daily parenting journey.

Your trust is the greatest reward I could ask for. Thank you for your dedication to the health and well-being of your children. May this book help you make every meal a joyful and nourishing experience.

I am very interested in what you think of this book.

Please leave a review on Amazon

or on my Facebook page:

The Magical World of Vita Kostiuk's Books
@magikwordvk

I will be very happy and grateful to you!

With love and gratitude!

www.ingramcontent.com/pod-product-compliance
Lightning Source LLC
Chambersburg PA
CBHW061051250726
48653CB00001B/356